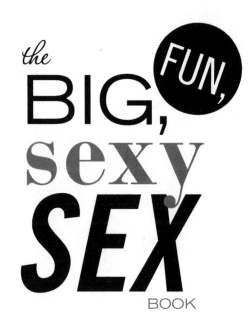

the
BIG, FUN,
sexy
SEX
BOOK

G

Gallery Books

NEW YORK

LONDON

TORONTO

SYDNEY

NEW DELHI

the BIG, *FUN,* sexy SEX BOOK

LISA RINNA & IAN KERNER, PH.D.

Gallery Books
A Division of Simon & Schuster, Inc.
1230 Avenue of the Americas
New York, NY 10020

First Gallery Books hardcover edition May 2012

GALLERY BOOKS and colophon are registered trademarks of Simon & Schuster, Inc.

For information about special discounts for bulk purchases, please contact Simon & Schuster Special Sales at 1-866-506-1949 or business@simonandschuster.com.

The Simon & Schuster Speakers Bureau can bring authors to your live event. For more information or to book an event contact the Simon & Schuster Speakers Bureau at 1-866-248-3049 or visit our website at www.simonspeakers.com.

Designed by Jaime Putorti

Manufactured in the United States of America

10 9 8 7 6 5 4 3 2

Library of Congress Cataloging-in-Publication Data is on file.

ISBN 978-1-4516-6123-1
ISBN 978-1-4516-6124-8 (ebook)

To our inspiring spouses,

Lisa Rubisch and *Harry Hamlin:*

for better, for worse,

for love and for life!

contents

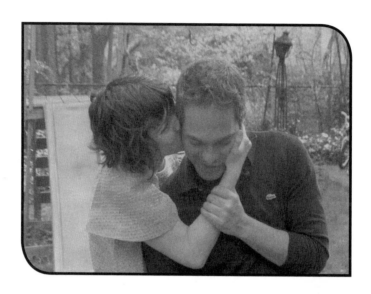

What happens outside the bedroom affects what happens in the bedroom, and when couples are connected intimately, their relationship can be more vital and stronger than they ever imagined.

—Ian Kerner

As a Hollywood actress, I know better than anyone that we live in a culture that slavishly worships youth, and where real women are gradually stripped of their sexual power. But don't underestimate a real woman. You want to see sexy? I'll show you sexy! You want to know about great sex? I'll show you great sex. You want a cougar? I'll give you a tigress! I'm just reaching my peak, and I feel sexier than ever—and so can you!

—Lisa Rinna

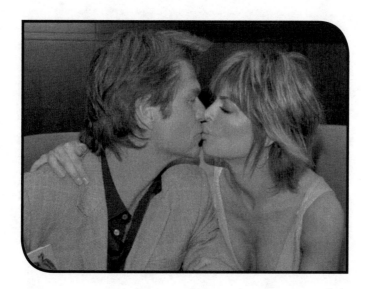

Harry Hamlin and I are two actors who have been together for twenty years. That's like 150 in Hollywood years! And honestly, sex—and by that I mean great sex—is a big part of what keeps us together and strong.

—Lisa Rinna

the
BIG, FUN,
sexy
SEX
BOOK

INTRODUCTION

We believe that sex matters—your sex life in particular!

Sex is the glue that binds couples together. It's what makes us more than just friends. Without sex, lovers become roommates, and a bedroom becomes just a place to sleep. Without sex, life has no . . . *life*.

Sure, being comfortable and cozy in your relationship is great. You can finish each other's sentences, love and accept his extra ten pounds, and know just how to satisfy each other in bed (or at least think you do). But too much comfort can also be challenging to your sex life:

- Have flannel PJs replaced your silky negligees?

- Are you more likely to nod off cradling the remote—instead of your partner?

- Are you too tired for sex?

- Is foreplay becoming "boreplay"?

A sex life is a terrible thing to waste. According to CNN, more than forty million Americans are stuck in sexless marriages, and according to a survey by Durex, more than 52 percent of us are dissatisfied with our love lives. Hey, it's only normal: After you've had sex with the same person at least a thousand times, it's easy to fall into a routine. You know each other's bodies and you know how to get where you're going, but as a couple you don't know how to appreciate the journey anymore. Where once your sex life was running on a full tank of anticipation and desire, suddenly the "near empty" light is flashing.

You probably didn't mean for it to get this way: Maybe you were planning to stop and fill the tank, but got distracted. Or maybe you took desire for granted. Whatever the reasons—whether you're frazzled by the demands of work and parenthood, or have simply grown too lazy to make an effort—sex is no longer a priority. And that's a problem. But no matter how dull, routine, or nonexistent your sex life seems now, it's never too late to reignite that spark. If your sex life's tank is empty, think of this book as fuel—rocket fuel! Whether you're seeking to solve a problem, learn a new technique, or dramatically improve your sex skills, we will help you take your sex life to the next level.

■ ■ ■

In these pages, you'll learn:

- The different libido types and how to align with your partner sexually

- What you need to do *outside* the bedroom to steam things up between the sheets

- Why great sex is good for you

- The best sexual positions for female orgasm

- How to spice up your sex life with new moves and tricks

- Oral sex and hand job tips guaranteed to drive a man wild

- How to push your sexual boundaries without embarrassment

- The best toys to turn you—and your partner—on

- Steamy role-playing scenarios that turn fantasies into reality

- The pros and cons of porn, and how to enjoy it with your partner

- How to cope with male and female sexual dysfunction

- Advice for keeping your sex life hot once you become a parent

- Why sex can get better as you get older

- Lisa's nutrition and exercise program designed to help you "get your sexy back"

- Fun "sexercises" to help add new spark to sex

And much, much more. There's a whole world of sexual options to be explored—and we want to help you start expanding your horizons. So get comfortable, grab your partner, and get ready to start having some fun.

WHY WE WROTE THIS BOOK

We've made it our mission to help you reclaim a mind-blowing sex life—or perhaps achieve one for the first time. True, we seem quite different on the surface: Lisa is a Hollywood bombshell known for her TV and movie roles, flirty rhythms on *Dancing with the Stars,* and frank discussions about sex with Howard Stern. Ian is a New York City sex counselor who works with couples grappling with sexual issues and who aims to educate people about the ins and outs of sex through his books, blogs, and Good in Bed website (www.goodinbed.com). Yet we both have a lot in common, too: We're both in long-term relationships—Lisa has been married to actor Harry Hamlin for nearly twenty years, and Ian just celebrated his tenth anniversary with his wife, also named Lisa. We have two children each—Lisa has two daughters, and Ian has two sons. We both understand what it's like to be with one person for a long time and how your relationship—and sex life—can change once you become a parent. We know how amazing sex can be, but we're also all too familiar with the struggles every couple goes through to keep things fun and fresh.

Because we're both so much on the same page (literally!), we wrote this book as a team, with the information and advice in the main text coming from both of us. Sometimes, one of us has something especially personal or unique to share; you'll find those stories in separate sidebars throughout the book.

LISA'S STORY

Why did I decide to write a book about sex? Believe me, I ask myself that every day! If you had asked me even just a few years ago if I thought I would someday write about such a personal subject, I would have blushed, laughed—and told you that you were crazy. But in my first book, *Rinnavation,* I spoke candidly about my personal struggles with postpartum depression as well as my loss of desire and subsequent search to put the sizzle back into my marriage. That section of the book led women to approach me wherever I went, asking me for ways that they, too, could put the "sex" back in their sex lives.

As I'll share in these pages, though, I haven't always felt sexually confident. My journey to a satisfying sex life has taken me from a series of unhealthy relationships to a wonderful marriage with my husband, Harry. But I didn't get here on my own. Along the way, I've consulted friends, therapists, "sexperts," pole-dancing instructors, and even Howard Stern! And what I've learned is this: It doesn't matter how hot you look; it matters how hot you feel. Sexiness and sensuality come from within, and there's no more powerful aphrodisiac than confidence. Being sexual means being vibrant, being alive, and being comfortable in your own skin. Sexuality is a vital life force, but too many women have lost touch with their own inner sense of eros, or life has chipped away at their sense of sexual self-esteem. Too many women "want to want" sex, but just don't. And they've stopped trying. And that's a shame: for them, and for their partner. Having a sex drive means just that—being driven: *driven* to take charge of one's sexuality, *driven* to try new things, and *driven* to be in the sort of relationship that supports having great sex.

That's the biggest lesson I want to share with you, and it's why I decided to write this book with Ian. Both as an expert and a man, he understands how sex works in the real world—when you've got a job, kids, a busy life. And he knows how important it is to feel self-assured in—and out of—bed. All the sex tips in the world don't matter much if you don't have the confidence to back them up.

IAN'S STORY

As a sex counselor, I spend a lot of time working with couples to help them achieve better sex lives. Some of them are coping with a sexual issue such as premature ejaculation, erectile disorder, or arousal problems, but many are simply trying to match up with their partner sexually. These days, that's tougher than ever, with crazy schedules, the distractions of modern technology, and preoccupations with pornography all conspiring to play havoc with a couple's sex life. As a result, a lot of couples find themselves leading lives of quiet desperation: Each person wants to feel more sexually open and free with the other, but—whether because of embarrassment, laziness, or fear—neither one speaks up.

I think a lot of this is because many people still feel uncomfortable talking about sex, even if they're already having it with each other. It's kind of silly when you think about it: Couples talk about all sorts of difficult, serious issues, from child care, to financial woes, to health crises. Yet somehow, when it comes to sex, we blush and bite our tongues—even if those tongues have already spent a lot of time exploring each other!

Shouldn't sex be fun? Shouldn't talking about sex be, well, sexy? I may be a clinician, but I believe that sex should be anything but clinical. So does Lisa, which is why I'm thrilled to have her as my coauthor. I think you'll find her frank, "game for anything" approach contagious—she's living proof that with the right attitude, it's never too late to get the sex life you've always wanted. That's the spirit with which Lisa and I have approached writing this book, and that's the spirit with which we want you to approach your relationship, both inside and outside the bedroom.

My daughters are far too young for explicit sex information like this right now. But I hope that when they're adults, they'll feel as empowered about their sexuality as I've come to feel about mine. I want them—and you—to know just how satisfying sex can be, especially when it's part of a loving, spiritual, committed relationship. Since rediscovering my own lost libido (and then some), I've been on a mission to inspire women everywhere to live their love lives to the fullest. My hope in this book is not just to give you some really great tips and techniques for making love to your guy but to help you unleash your sexual self-esteem and be your sexiest self regardless of your age. If Ian and I can help you to feel stronger, more sensual, and more playful, we'll have done our jobs. And you'll enjoy a vibrant sex life, too.

If you come away from reading this book with anything, we hope that it's the ability to communicate with your partner comfortably about sex, and a new sense of playfulness and joy. We've called this *The Big, Fun, Sexy Sex Book,* after all!

So let's have some fun!

part one

·

OUTSIDE
the
BEDROOM

before you can get in sync with your partner inside the bedroom, you've got to get in sync *outside* the bedroom. But that's not always so easy: One or both of you may be stressed about work, money, family, or any number of factors. Maybe you feel overwhelmed or exhausted and sex is the last thing on your mind. Or maybe you're dealing with nonsexual relationship issues (whether it's bickering or more serious concerns) that still play havoc with your sex life. Remember, the brain is our biggest sex organ, and when you're not satisfied with other aspects of your relationship, you're probably not going to be very satisfied with sex.

Of course, we all know That Couple—the one that fights constantly like cats and dogs right in front of you. The one that always seems on the verge of a breakup. The one that, according to your friend, has amazing sex that keeps her coming back for more, even if the guy is bad for her (and vice versa). Maybe you've even been in such a relationship yourself: one that was wrong in most aspects but sexually exciting. In fact, it's that kind of mind-blowing sex that makes some otherwise unhappy couples justify staying together. It begs the question: Is the quality or health of a relationship *really* connected to a couple's sexual satisfaction?

The answer is a resounding "absolutely"! And that's not just lip service. Research has shown that the happiest relationships are also the most sexually satisfying relationships over the long term. You can have a bad relationship with amazing sex, but that satisfaction rarely lasts. These relationships either don't endure over the long term or they become less satisfying—and, eventually, the sex follows suit. Sure, some people love the passion of angry sex. And we'll admit, there is something to be said for the thrill of makeup sex. In general, though, relationship conflict and good sex go together about as well as oil and water. Over time, the cycle of fighting can take its toll on one or both of you, and the excitement of all that great sex ebbs.

The truth is, it's tough for many of us to feel sexy when we're upset. Anger can lead to low sexual desire, especially if resentment and hostility have been simmering for a while. Negative feelings can also interfere with arousal, so even if you think you want sex, your body might not agree. It can be difficult to relax and respond sexually when you're feeling angry, hurt, sad, or otherwise upset: Women may experience vaginal dryness or painful intercourse, while men may have trouble getting an erection or may find it more difficult to ejaculate. The mind plays a crucial role in sexual function, and your body just might not respond when you don't feel comfortable, connected, or safe. It's not surprising that Ian and other sex experts find that when a sexual complaint crops up in a relationship, such as low desire, there's often a nonsexual relationship issue behind it.

Even if your relationship is strong, outside factors can also put a damper on sexual desire, arousal, and function. And between work, personal obligations, and relationships with family and friends—especially if you're caring for children or aging parents—stress is everywhere. Add in worries about the economy, your health, your pets, even that little mildew problem in the shower that you've been ignoring, and you can see why little stressors can combine to create big sex hurdles. There's no doubt about it—what goes on in between your ears can have a huge impact on what goes on between the sheets.

Stress is a part of life, and ups and downs are part of any long-term relationship. If something's "off" in one aspect of your world, it's likely that your sex life will be out of whack, too. Fortunately, there's a lot you can do to help your relationship—and your libido—thrive. Even simple acts like hugging each other or doing the dishes can go a long way toward your satisfaction, in and out of bed. So get ready to discover how to maximize your relationship in the bedroom by putting in some effort everywhere else.

POP QUIZ

According to a recent study by Trojan, how many times a year does the average American adult have sex?

(A) 365 **(B)** 84 **(C)** 26.4 **(D)** 7

Correct Answer: (B) 84. That's more than once a week, which isn't bad for the average couple. When you go more than a week without sex, you become vulnerable to sex ruts and all the relationship problems that go along with a slump. If you're not having sex once a week with your partner, it might be a question of making time for sex and pushing it to the top of your to-do list.

1

MAKING THE CONNECTION

In part 2 of this book, we'll talk about the biochemistry responsible for, well, your chemistry. In short, feelings of lust, love, and newness boost your brain's production of the neurotransmitter dopamine, which in turn triggers feelings of pleasure and satisfaction. The downside of dopamine: Levels tend to return to normal after the novelty of a new lover wears off—about two years into a relationship.

That's the plight of every long-term couple, but it doesn't mean that you're doomed to spend the rest of your life stuck in a boring (or sexless) relationship. Research shows that dopamine isn't the only chemical messenger affected by love, and it isn't the only one required to keep relationships strong. In one study, researchers scanned the brains of older volunteers who claimed to still be in love after twenty years of marriage. They found that not only did some lucky subjects still have higher levels of dopamine, but the long-term couples also had higher levels of oxytocin, a feel-good brain chemical (called a neurotransmitter) linked to a sense of emotional intimacy, relaxation, attachment and bonding, contentment, and trust. That makes sense, since other research suggests that this "cuddle hormone" can help foster loving relationships: A 2009 study published in *Biological Psychiatry* found couples who received a spray form of oxytocin before an argument showed more positive and less negative behavior than those who were given a placebo. Oxytocin also appears to help relieve stress, improve mood, and lower blood pressure.

With benefits like these, it's no wonder that we could all use some more oxytocin. Fortunately, that's pretty easy—and enjoyable—to achieve, particularly for women, who produce higher amounts of the chemical. You've also got more opportunities to raise your levels: Childbirth, breastfeeding, and orgasm all trigger its release. Of course, having and nursing a baby, while wonderful, isn't an experience you can (or would want to) repeat continually. And, as much as we'd love it to be otherwise, nonstop orgasms just aren't realistic.

Instead, getting a daily boost of oxytocin is within your grasp—literally. Nonsexual touch can also increase levels: Studies even show that just a twenty- to thirty-second hug can raise oxytocin levels in both men and women. (Women may benefit even more, since the female hormone estrogen appears to intensify oxytocin.) So make it a point to hug each other at least three times today, for at least thirty seconds at a time. Thirty seconds may seem almost uncomfortably long—at first, you may find yourselves giggling self-consciously, making jokes, and wondering how much time has passed. And some guys will end up checking

lisa says . . . HUG IT OUT

I love hugging Harry—and being hugged by him. (After all, those hunky arms were one of the first things I noticed about him when we first met!) I can't lie, though: Thirty seconds can seem like an awfully long time when you first start embracing, and if you're like me, your brain will naturally start going to all those things you could be doing instead, from helping the kids with their homework to running errands. Don't give in to those thoughts! Fight to keep yourself in the moment. I like to focus on the way Harry's body feels against mine and remember all the things I love about him, but you should do whatever works for you. Before you know it, those thirty seconds will have passed—and you'll both feel so good that you'll be craving another hit of oxytocin. Pretty soon, those long, loving hugs will become second nature.

their watches. Hang in there: It gets easier, and the results are worth it. Both of us practice these thirty-second hugs with our spouses, and love how they seem to create a bond that lasts throughout the day—and night.

RELATIONSHIP SLUMPS: ACCENTUATE THE POSITIVE

Oxytocin-boosting hugs are just one example of what's called "transferable desire." Forget the clunky name—basically, it means all those little nonsexual connections that you and your partner make outside the bedroom. Without those crucial connections, you're more likely to fall into the dreaded relationship slump. And if you've ever felt out of sync with your partner in other ways, you've probably seen the effects of this disharmony sexually, too. When you've been with your partner for a long time, it's easy to start to devalue and disregard each other, and when that happens, neither one of you is going to want sex. We believe this is one reason why so many people find themselves in sexless marriages: When you're not feeling the love, why would you want to *make* love? If you've been in a slump long enough, you begin to wonder if your relationship is even worth saving.

The good news, thankfully, is that with a little work and a lot of patience, you can prevent that slump from turning into a total collapse. It all starts with what Lisa has dubbed "HER": Hyperawareness, Effort, and Responsibility.

You've got to be *hyperaware* of your partner and the state of your relationship: Watch for negativity and that devaluing we mentioned earlier, and give your partner the respect he deserves.

All relationships require *effort*: You've both got to put the time and energy into each other to thrive, whether that means giving him extra attention, asking for the same in return, or both.

And *responsibility* is crucial: As much as you may want to believe in Prince Charming, you just can't rely on your man to magically "fix" everything in your relationship. It usually takes two people to dig themselves into a rut, and it takes two of you to crawl out. When you change the way you do things, you change the way your partner responds to you.

If that rut seems especially deep, we're certainly in favor of getting help from a third party. No, not a threesome! (It should go without saying, but if you're already sinking, adding another person to the mix isn't going keep you afloat.) We're talking about couples counseling, which can help you move past obstacles and give your relationship a jump start. Therapy doesn't mean you're doomed as a couple—in fact, it shows that you're willing to do the work necessary to succeed. As Lisa says, "Harry and I have no problem visiting a therapist from time to time if we think it will help. We think relationships are a lot like gardens—sometimes you've just got to get in there and do some weeding!"

Whether or not you pursue couples therapy, there's a lot you can do to get out of a rut and back on track. In a lot of cases, all it takes is some positivity. In fact, studies show that the most successful relationships tend to have a high ratio of positive to negative interactions. Ian is a fan of couples counselor Dr. John Gottman, who believes that this ratio should be five to one: five positive interactions (hugging, holding hands, having a positive conversation) for every negative one (bickering, for example). If you're interested in reading more about Dr. Gottman's work, check out his book *The Seven Principles for Making Marriage Work,* which outlines tips for reinforcing the positive aspects of relationships.

Of course, you can't go through life tallying every interaction, but you probably already have a pretty good sense of whether the good in your relationship outweighs the not so good. So think about it: Do you hold hands while walking through the supermarket? Lean into each other as you watch your favorite show together? Cook a meal or clean up together afterward? All these "little things" really do add up over time. And while they may not seem sexual, they create a surplus of transferable desire that helps fuel sexual desire. Simply put, if things are going well in your relationship out of bed, you're more likely to want to get *into* bed together.

One way to help you focus on the positive is to remember what attracted you to your partner in the first place. For instance, perhaps you were attracted by the fact that your partner had a nice build, was a great cook, and had a scathing sense of humor. Now think about which of those things are still true. There may also be a few new positive attributes you could add to the list—maybe he's a wonderful, attentive parent to your child or is willing to give you regular foot massages. Of course, there will probably also be some negative attributes: He's a total slob or doesn't like to socialize with your friends, for example. Make a list of both those positive and negative attributes.

Now, looking at your lists of positive and negative attributes, think about how the negatives have gotten in the way of experiencing the positives. It would certainly be nice if your partner magically transformed himself into the perfect dream man. Sorry to burst your bubble, but chances are that's not going to happen. So try to imagine situations where his negative tendency or attribute might not come into play, or situations that bring out the positive. Let's say that when you and your partner go out, the fact that he's slob becomes less of an obstacle to your enjoyment, since you're not in situations where he can be messy. Or maybe you're able to best enjoy your partner on one-on-one dates, rather than forcing him to hang out with your friends.

Finished? Now create a short list of simple situations that give your positive feelings about your guy a chance to flourish: date nights that get you out of the house and away from his piles of dirty laundry, for example, or thirty-second hugs that let you revel in his strong arms. When you and your partner work to bring out the best in each other, you're more apt to respect each other, less prone to bickering—and way more likely to get that oxytocin flowing. Novelty and newness, on the other hand, can help increase dopamine, so experimenting with anything different—whether that's wearing a new piece of lingerie, trying out a new sexual position, or pretending to be strangers on a first date—can replenish levels of this neurotransmitter, as you'll learn later on.

Let's talk for a moment about another way that you can recapture that excitement that was so strong when you first met. It's simple, really: You want to be able to foster the sense of mystery that makes new relationships so hot while still

good idea: LITTLE THINGS MEAN A LOT

For many couples, negative interactions take far less effort than positive ones. Don't believe us? Think about how easy it is to bicker about meaningless stuff—you might not even realize you're doing it until after the fact. Now consider the following activities. How often do you and your partner engage in *these* on a weekly basis?

- Hug/embrace
- Hold hands
- Kiss
- Say I love you
- Call during the day to say hi and check in
- Compliment each other
- E-mail each other
- Eat meals together
- Take time to really talk about each other's day
- Do chores together
- Go on regular date nights
- Watch favorite TV shows or read the newspaper together
- Socialize with other people together
- Cultivate/participate in mutual hobbies/ common interests
- Go on vacations together

If you engage in at least half of these activities, a few times a week or more, you're probably connected on an emotional level. If not, try to think about ways to increase the frequency of positive interactions in your daily life. You'll be surprised how easy it is once you get started.

enjoying the intimacy, comfort, and dependability that go hand in hand with long-term love. And one of the easiest ways to do that is to look at the way you currently act around each other—and then compare that to the way you acted in the beginning. Don't get us wrong. We think feeling comfortable is a good thing. In fact, women tend to *need* that sense of comfort to be able to relax and let go in bed. There's such a thing, however, as feeling *too* comfortable around each other.

See, there's a fine line between comfort and laziness—the difference, say, between knowing the intricacies of your partner's body and knowing the intricacies of his bathroom habits. The very closeness most of us crave has a knack for acting like a heavy, wet blanket on attraction, snuffing out the sexual spark that often brings a couple together in the first place. So while you may consider your guy to be your "best friend"—and have no qualms about vegging out on the couch in your sweatpants or clipping your toenails in front of him—you probably also find yourself missing the unpredictability and mystery that defined the early days of your relationship. Which of the following bad habits are you and your partner guilty of?

- Sleep with kids or pets in your bed or bedroom

- Have (and use) a television, computer, or smartphone in your bedroom

- Spend your evenings surfing the Internet, e-mailing, visiting social networking sites, or playing computer games

- Bring your cell or smartphone on "date nights" or spend time texting or playing with your phone in your partner's presence

- Leave the door open while in the bathroom

- Perform personal grooming habits (flossing your teeth, clipping your nails, etc.) in front of your partner

- Sometimes skip basic hygiene (bathing, brushing your teeth, shaving, etc.) because you're too tired, lazy, or think your partner doesn't care

Now think back to the beginning of your relationship: Which of the previous acts would you have performed in front of your partner? Which would have made you feel embarrassed? By cutting out some of these vices, you can stay comfortable in your relationship while injecting back some of the spark and mystery.

ian says . . . PUT YOURSELVES FIRST

As one half of a married couple myself, I can't stress this enough: You've got to be selfish about your relationship. Couples have a lot of combined obligations and responsibilities, way more than you ever had as individuals: to children, to family and friends, and it's easy to put everyone else first as you try to maintain a master schedule. Don't stop putting your relationship first: from date nights to vacations to making time for each other, stay selfish. Think about the preflight safety instructions you hear on airplanes: You've got to secure your own oxygen mask before you can do the same for your child. Yet in many marriages, couples end up putting their kids before themselves, which can eventually suffocate your relationship with your partner—and impair your ability to parent well. So put on your own oxygen masks first, take a deep breath, and watch everyone in your life, especially your children, start breathing easier.

2

LIVING IN THE MOMENT

Picture this: You're in the heat of the moment and your guy looks deep into your eyes and whispers, "What are you thinking?" So what's your answer? We're willing to bet it's something along the lines of "Oh, nothing" or "Just about how sexy you are!" *Liar.* Yes, we said it—and we're probably right. If you're like most women, your brain just doesn't go blissfully blank, even in the throes of passion. Admit it: From work, to your kids, to your mother-in-law, to what to make for dinner tomorrow, to whether you're out of laundry detergent, you're probably thinking about anything and everything *except* sex.

Distracting? You bet. But also perfectly normal. If you've ever tried to meditate and failed, you know just how difficult it can be to stay in the moment. Now add all the pressure and excitement of sex, and you can see why it's easy to "lose" an orgasm just when it seems about to happen. Stress even affects your biochemistry: Levels of oxytocin decrease when you're tense. And that's a problem, since research has shown that women really need to feel relaxed during sex to let go and enjoy pleasure for pleasure's sake, even in new and exciting relationships. In this chapter, we'll show you how to do just that.

TALKING DIRTY: WHY CHOREPLAY IS THE NEW FOREPLAY

Ever seen a book called *Porn for Women*? The cover sports a smiling man performing an act that undoubtedly makes many women sigh with pleasure: He's vacuuming the living room. Inside the pages, another man does laundry, promising to go grocery shopping with the kids "so you can relax." Or consider the lyrics to "Might Get Lucky," from singer Darius Rucker: "I'll chase the kids around the yard all afternoon / Put away the dishes so she don't have to / Fix

lisa says . . . TAKE FIVE

To me, the gift of sex is simple: Good sex makes me happy, and when I feel happy, my life just seems better all around. It's pretty clear that we women also crave the intimacy and connection that sex offers. But as the main caretakers for our families (not to mention trying to also be the perfect wife, mother, daughter, and worker!), achieving the relaxed state we need to stay in that sexual moment can be a challenge.

That's why I think it's so important to take time for ourselves every day, even if it's just ten or twenty minutes. So ask your guy to help you get a little bit of alone time by taking care of the kids or helping out around the house. Don't feel guilty: This break will pay off later in the bedroom—for both of you. Here are five of my favorite ways to chill out.

■ **Get moving.** I've always been a big fan of exercise, whether that's taking a yoga or spin class, jogging, or dancing (at home with Harry and the kids, in a class, or even on TV with my amazing *Dancing with the Stars* partner, Louis Van Amstel). Ideally, you're already getting some regular exercise—as you'll learn in part 4 of this book, yoga and Pilates are especially important for great sex: They not only relieve stress and boost mood, they also tone and tighten the core muscles you use in bed! If you want to get calm quickly, though, a walk around the block or a few yoga-based stretches can work wonders.

the screen door on the porch like I said I'd do / And if I'm right on the money / You know I might get lucky."

Hmm. We think they just might be on to something! These pop culture offerings actually hit on what women—and experts—have known for years: If a guy wants some action, he needs to get his hands on a bottle of Windex before he gets them on you. When it comes to a satisfying sex life, "choreplay" is the new foreplay.

Choreplay doesn't, as one friend's partner suggested hopefully, involve you giving him some oral attention while he does the dishes—although we suppose

■ **Run a bath.** There's nothing like sinking into a tub of hot water to center your mind and ease tense muscles. Add some lavender-scented bath salts to relax even more. A hot shower with nice-smelling bath gel has similar effects. If you're lucky, your sweetie might even join you and offer to rub your back.

■ **Breathe deeply.** My great aesthetician, Susan Ciminelli, once shared this quick chill-out tip with me: Lightly press your forefinger and thumb together (this is said to create calming energy), close your eyes, and breathe deeply for three to eight minutes. The exercise is supposed to be the equivalent of eight hours of sleep. I don't know if that's true, but I practice it whenever I can—whether in the back of a cab or in line at the grocery store—and I swear it de-stresses me.

■ **Have a sip.** I certainly don't recommend relying on alcohol to cope with stress, but if you don't have a problem with dependency, there's nothing wrong with enjoying an occasional glass of wine to help unwind. I also find chamomile and other noncaffeinated teas to be very calming.

■ **Read a book.** Or a magazine. Or watch your favorite TV show, listen to music you enjoy, get a massage, go shopping (for yourself, not your family), or indulge in a mani/pedi. The key is to spend some time alone—even if it's just a few minutes—doing something that makes you feel good.

that's cool, too. Instead, choreplay is anything he does to help out around the house or with the kids. Ladies, we know you're all too familiar with this scenario: You come home from one job only to be burdened by a "second shift" of cleaning, cooking, and chaos that makes sex just one more task on your to-do list. The goal of choreplay is for your partner to move sex to the top of that list by helping you cross off some of the less scintillating items.

Choreplay is a hot topic in research circles these days, and a number of recent studies support its effectiveness as a form of foreplay. One recent study from the University of Western Ontario, for example, found that wives are happier when their husbands pitch in with housework. Another report from researchers at the University of Illinois at Chicago even suggests men who help clean, take care of their kids, and do other domestic chores may see the benefits of their labor pay off in the bedroom.

Of course, it's no secret that men aren't mind readers, but most of them are aware enough to notice when the sink is full of dishes or the garbage is overflowing. But unless he's a sex counselor like Ian—or *really* into housework—he may not understand the connection between, say, Scrubbing Bubbles and sex. You're probably going to have to explain the concept of choreplay to your man—and even then, you may need to be explicit about handing over some tasks to him. There's a fine line between asking and nagging, however. Take a tip from Lisa, who has no qualms about asking her husband to lend a hand. "You can ask a man to pitch in without browbeating him," she says. "It's okay to exaggerate a bit: Make him feel like he's a hero and that you really need his help." If your guy needs encouragement, remind him that men who take care of their kids are sexy—and that a clean house can help put you in the mood.

Tension Tamer

Still having trouble letting go and living in the sexual moment? You're not alone. A study published in the October 2010 issue of the *Journal of Sexual Medicine* found that among women who reported having low sexual desire, 60 percent cited stress or fatigue as a reason. That's a shame, since other research shows that sex itself helps reduce stress: In one 2007 study published in the *Archives of Sexual Behavior*, researchers found that having sex or even simply being affectionate with a partner was linked to a better mood and lower stress the following day.

Clearly, it's time to start giving yourself some more attention. That may sound counterintuitive: Isn't the problem that you're already too wrapped up in your own mind? Well, yes. But the key to really relaxing is to unwind before you even get between those sheets. First, though, think about whether you're truly in the mood for sex tonight. If you've had a tough day, feel exhausted, or have got other things on your mind, there's no reason to push things. Temporarily putting sex on the back burner can allow you and your partner to focus on what you need to get done, or on finding quiet moments to regroup. Sex will still be there tomorrow!

If it seems like you're constantly stressed or feeling disconnected and distracted during sex, though, it's time to take things into your own hands and figure out what you can do to chill out. Once you start relaxing outside of bed, it's easier to stay in that sexual moment *in* bed. So learn to let go. You're going to need your full attention for the bedroom tricks coming up in part 5!

try this: FEATHER YOUR LOVE NEST

After you've had sex with the same person over and over, it's easy to fall into a routine: You fall asleep watching TV or give each other a quick peck on the lips before bed.

Want to get your groove back? Try giving your boudoir a little makeover. It's time to declutter your bedroom and add inspiration—think scented candles and sexy music—that heightens the senses and promotes deep relaxation. You're going spice things up by transforming your humble bedroom into a love nest. In fact, the very act of preparing your bedroom can act as a sort of extended foreplay by building even more anticipation of just what will happen in that room later on.

Don't worry if you're on a budget. While you may need a trip or two to the store for some supplies, much of your decorating will involve re-purposing what you've already got. Here's how:

■ First, ask yourself what you'd think if you were about to make love to your partner in this room after seeing it for the first time. Does the ambience put you in the mood? Or does the pile of laundry in the corner make you want to run screaming in the other direction?

■ Now clear out that clutter! Leaving it there will only distract you from more important things—like sex. Socks, piles of magazines, dead houseplants—give it all the old heave-ho.

■ Now, consider what's left. Could you use some new sheets? What about the colors in the room? (Pale blues and greens are ideal for relaxation, which is crucial for female desire, but you should also add pops of red and pink in order to turn up the heat on your love life. Bring in some throw pillows from the living room or a rug from your guest bedroom, for example.) Consider repainting the room, or even just altering the color palette with accent pillows, a new bedspread, or colored lights. Freshen up the room's smell with fresh flowers or candles scented with cinnamon and vanilla, which have been shown to increase arousal and attraction. Don't forget to make a sexy playlist of songs that turn you on, then hook up your CD player or iPod.

■ Now get yourself a "toy box," whether it's a Rubbermaid container or a carved wooden chest. Fill it with adults-only playthings such as massage oils and massage candles (special candles containing scented wax that when melted acts as a moisturizing massage cream), personal lubricant, honey dust, vibrating toys . . . anything that appeals to you and your partner. (If you have kids, be sure to use a box with a lock and keep it out of reach.) You're going to have lots of opportunities to enjoy your sexy new bedroom, especially when you follow the tips in the rest of this book!

part two

·

WHAT'S YOUR (sex) TYPE?

You say to-*may*-to, he says to-*mah*-to. You're an Aquarius, he's a Leo. You're the life of the party, his idea of the perfect evening involves his La-Z-Boy and the Lakers. Yet somehow, you make it work. You're not alone: Few of us have everything in common with our partners—and that's just fine. After all, who wants to look and act exactly alike? (Well, maybe those couples who tend to wear matching outfits—but frankly, we find that kind of creepy.) Those individual attributes that make you unique are an intrinsic part of what attracted you to each other in the first place.

The truth is, once you're in a relationship with someone, you tend to accept such variations and find common ground. Maybe you're a Democrat and he's a Republican, for example, but you share the same penchant for wry, sarcastic humor or you enjoy engaging in lighthearted political banter over your favorite bottle of Pinot. Or maybe you're like Lisa and her husband, Harry, whose very different upbringings and demeanors (she's a sassy small-town girl; he's a more reserved Ivy Leaguer) make them appear polar opposites on the surface, but whose mutual respect and commitment to each other actually make them a perfect fit. Or maybe you're like Ian and his wife, Lisa, who look a lot alike on the outside (small, dark hair, blue eyes—they've even been referred to as twins), but couldn't be more different on the inside (she's optimistic and glass half full and he's cynical and, well, drinking straight from the bottle). While it may not be true that opposites attract, they at least keep life interesting.

In fact, research suggests that when it comes to staying together, your overall approach to life may matter more than your specific differences: One study of 291 married couples, published in the February 2005 issue of the *Journal of Personality and Social Psychology,* found that similar personalities were more important than similarities in attitude, religion, and values in predicting a happy relationship. The bottom line: You don't have to be mirror images of each other to have a successful relationship.

But what happens when your differences occur between the sheets? If you're sexually incompatible, you probably didn't realize it for a while. In fact, you might have felt like your bodies were made for each other. Great sexual chemistry is undeniable—and obvious to almost everyone. (Go rent *Mr. and Mrs. Smith* or any film with Spencer Tracy and Katharine Hepburn and try to tell us we're wrong!) And when you're in those first heady stages of a new romance, it's so easy to get caught up in all that heart-pounding giddiness of excitement and attraction. That's because, in the beginning of your relationship, you've both been hijacked by a potent neurochemical cocktail of infatuation hormones that's responsible for your constant canoodling—that wonderful "can't keep your hands off each other" phase that many long-term couples desperately yearn to re-create. Your new coupledom itself is so novel and thrilling that all you need is love (and sex!).

There is, of course, a downside to infatuation: Just as it tends to distract you from those irritating little traits that later become larger annoyances—leaving the toilet seat up, snoring, watching the Sox game out of the corner of his eye during a date—it also masks more troubling differences in the bedroom. Simply put, you're so busy getting busy that you probably won't notice potential sexual incompatibility until your infatuation starts to wane.

Eventually, though, those hormones start to ebb—and you begin to discover that your seemingly hot sex life might not really be so smokin'. Maybe he turns the lights on during sex but you switch them right back off. Or maybe he wants to do it in the restroom of your local Starbucks but you get skittish anywhere outside the safety and comfort of your own bed. Maybe you crave sex every day, but he's perfectly content with doing it once a month. Or perhaps you love to talk about sex, while the very word makes him blush. And even if you do both like to get daring sexually, you and your partner may not always agree on what you'd like to try. As a new survey by Ian's website, Good in Bed, suggests, couples not only vary in their capacity for adventure, they also differ in which adventures—from watching porn together to adding a third person to the mix—appeal to them.

So do disparities such as these mean you're doomed to break up? Not necessarily. Sure, it can be disappointing to realize that you may not be sexually compatible. But it happens to the best of us. And, as you'll learn in this section, it's completely possible for sexually incompatible couples to have very compatible—and very steamy—relationships.

POP QUIZ

According to the World Health Organization, how many acts of sex occur every day around the world?

(A) 40 million   (B) 100 million   (C) 500 million   (D) 2 billion

Correct Answer: (B) 100 million. That's a lot of sexual activity, and yet—according to a recent report from CNN—more than 40 million Americans say they're stuck in sexless marriages. So clearly we need to get that total number to 140 million!

3

THE CHEMISTRY BEHIND YOUR CHEMISTRY

We've all been there: The butterflies in the stomach. The rush of attraction. The thrilling roller coaster ride of new love. And we all think the same thing: No one else has ever felt like *this* before! Well, we hate to break the news, but you're not the only couple to experience those frisky feelings. In fact, that initial exhilaration has less to do with Cupid's arrow and more to do with biochemical reactions. Of course, being smitten isn't solely the result of our biology—a sense of humor, nice legs, and smooth bedroom moves definitely help spark attraction. But that ecstatic, weak-in-the-knees sensation that accompanies a new relationship? That's mostly hormonal. Hot stuff, huh?

It's often been said that the brain really is our biggest sex organ. And that's never truer than when we first fall in love or, more accurately, lust. It works like this: When you're head over heels, activity increases in areas of your brain associated with intense romantic feelings, triggering increased levels of a neurotransmitter (or chemical messenger) called dopamine. This brain chemical is responsible for all kinds of good stuff like pleasure, satisfaction, elation, and greater energy—no wonder love is so grand! And the more romantic you feel, the higher your dopamine spikes. Dopamine is also linked to our reward center, meaning that not only does it trigger good feelings, it makes us crave more of them. Turns out we really are addicted to love.

But don't just take our word for it. There have been a number of studies on the effect of love and lust on the brain, with intriguing results. In one 2003 report by the Society for Neuroscience, researchers scanned the brains of seventeen young men and women while they looked at photos of people they loved and of people they knew but felt neutral about. They found increased dopamine activity in the brain regions linked to romantic love, as well as in a region shown to light up when people eat chocolate (as good a reason as any to indulge in some Godiva with your sweetie). The same study showed that love affects men's and women's brains differently: Most of the women had higher activity in areas associated with emotion, while most of the guys had higher activity in areas related to sexual activity. That's not to say that women don't feel horny when they're in love or that guys are only focused on sex rather than romance, but it does highlight some interesting differences in the way men and women feel and act, which we'll be discussing in more detail later on.

Other research on the science of attraction suggests that lust may be fleeting, but that long-term relationships have their own biological basis. When researchers at the University of Pisa in Italy tested blood levels of hormones called neutrophins in volunteers, they found that these brain chemicals were much higher in people who were in the early stages of romance. The sex hormone testosterone also increased in women—but decreased in men—who were in love. Similar studies have found that another chemical, called nerve growth factor, rises with romantic attraction as well. Yet two years into a relationship, all of these "love molecules" return to normal levels, confirming our fears that passion really does ebb after those initial sparks. The good news? Stable relationships can foster oxytocin, the glue that binds strong couples together—in and out of the bedroom. The challenge is to inject some novelty back into your stable relationship so that you can both enjoy higher levels of dopamine, too.

quick study: SNIFFING OUT COMPATIBILITY

When it comes to love and attraction, should you follow your nose? Maybe, according to recent research. Two large studies led by Brown University olfactory expert Dr. Rachel Herz found that women rank a man's scent as the most important feature for determining whether she would be interested in him sexually.

That's not surprising, since the genes that make up our immune system help determine our smell: Like fingerprints, each of us has our own unique "odor print," which is part of a region of genes known as the major histocompatibility complex (MHC). In another study, a wide variety of men were each asked to wear the same T-shirt for two days in a row, after which the shirts were put into identical boxes. Women were then asked to smell the shirts and to indicate which they thought would have the most sexually attractive wearers, based on the smell. The results showed that women were most attracted to men with an MHC most dissimilar from their own, while T-shirts worn by guys with similar MHC profiles tended to be rated as "fatherly" or "brotherly" but not sexually attractive. And a survey conducted by the research firm Strategy One found that 56 percent of women said they wouldn't date a guy who smells like their dad. So when we say that opposites attract, we may not be talking about differences in personality, but rather differences in immune systems. This is one of Nature's ways of ensuring that we produce the healthiest offspring. No wonder that a woman's sense of smell is at its peak when she's ovulating and most likely to get pregnant. Also, scent can trigger powerful memories, especially from our childhoods, which is why these scents may still exert a hold on us years later. And according to Dr. Alan Hirsch, director of the Smell & Taste Treatment and Research Foundation, "Research has shown that when women are in the presence of a preferred scent, they are more likely to project positive feelings on those around them, which can lead to increased attraction."

So lean in and take a good sniff of your guy—even if your libidos aren't always in sync, his scent may still make you compatible!

4

THE MATCH GAME: YOUR LIBIDO TYPE

We know what you're thinking: *That biology lesson was great, guys, but what happens when those love molecules fade? Suddenly I've got a man who would rather read the latest* New Yorker *and give me the same old, same old than read erotic poetry and get all* 9½ Weeks *with me.*

We feel your pain. But here's the deal: You've likely *always* had a guy who preferred literary fiction and the missionary position—you were just too gaga over him to notice. He hasn't changed, and neither have you: Your hormones have. For couples who share the same sex style, this shift is no big deal. But when you feel like your dashing sex machine of a man has been replaced by Al Bundy (or, on the flip side, your sweet, cuddly charmer has morphed into Oscar the Grouch), well, you've got a problem.

Mismatched libidos—discrepancies in both what you like sexually and how often you like it—are a major issue for many couples and could help explain why an estimated forty million Americans are stuck in sex-starved marriages. And if you believe experts who say that there are many different types and subtypes of libidos, you can understand why it's so easy to not even be in the same book, let alone on the same page, as your partner.

While not everyone agrees on the number and characteristics of different libi-dos, it's clear that there's more than a one-size-fits-all approach to sex. According to sex therapist Sandra Pertot, Ph.D., there are ten main libido "types" that determine our sexual needs, desires, and expectations. We think the categories she's created—from the "erotic" libido type that craves intense, passionate love-making, to the "disinterested" lover with a lower sex drive—can be very helpful for sorting out some cases of mismatched libidos. If you and your partner seem to be light-years away from each other in bed, we recommend checking out Dr. Pertot's book on the subject, *When Your Sex Drives Don't Match*.

Not all cases of sexual incompatibility may be so complex, though. In Ian's experience working with couples, he's found that most of us lean toward one of two main libido groups: *thrill seekers* and *comfort creatures*. These categories are just what they sound like—they describe how much of a risk taker you are, sexu-ally speaking. Thrill seekers require a lot of novelty, and comfort creatures are much more content with a familiar bed. Don't get us wrong: Comfort creatures are anything but boring, and being a thrill seeker doesn't mean you're destined to cheat—in fact, many people with this libido type are happily monogamous. You might also assume that most men are thrill seekers and most women are comfort creatures. There's a bit of truth to this, probably because it's easier for most men to have an orgasm. For women, though, orgasms can be less consis-tent. Once you're having good sex with your partner, you don't usually want to change that. Why mess with a good thing? That's not always the case, though, and plenty of women do consider themselves thrill seekers. (Just ask Lisa, who

ian says . . .

I may be a sex counselor, but my own sex life is pretty ordinary. Don't get me wrong—my relationship with my wife is amazing. But if you think my line of work automatically means that we like to visit swingers' clubs or have mirrors on the ceiling of our bedroom, think again. Sexually speaking, my wife and I are both comfort creatures, and that suits us just fine.

considers herself something of a risk taker, both in and out of bed!) And you can't always predict whether your lover will be a thrill seeker or a comfort creature based on his profession, either: Ian may be a sex counselor but he is a confirmed comfort creature, for example.

Just as you can differ from your partner in what kind of sex you want, you can differ in how often you want it. Some people get antsy if they go more than a few days without sex, while others are perfectly happy doing the deed far less often. There's a stereotype that men always want sex more than women, but the truth is that they can be just as likely as you to offer up the old "not tonight, dear, I've got a headache" excuse. In fact, research suggests that about 20 to 30 percent of women and 10 to 20 percent of men say they have low sexual desire, an issue we'll talk about more in parts 9 and 10 of this book.

It stands to reason that sex is a bit simpler when you're with someone who has the same sex drive and libido type as you: Two comfort creatures are perfectly content to settle into bed for a sexy session that plays on everything they already know about each other's desire—a healthy helping of "if it ain't broke, don't fix it." They tend to prefer to keep sex within the comfort of their own homes, sticking to a few tried-and-true positions and routines. Two thrill seekers, on the other hand, can make the perfect partners in crime for a frisky hookup anywhere *but* the bedroom, dabbling in the latest sexual positions or toys along the way.

Things get a tad trickier when you find yourself in a relationship with a guy who's far more—or less—adventurous than you. If he seems disinterested in trying new things, you might start to feel bored. And if he's always looking for the latest, greatest sexual thrill, you might worry that you're not exciting enough for him and that *he's* losing interest. Sexual boredom is a very common problem in many relationships and can result in misunderstandings, confusion, hurt feelings, bruised egos, and—if you fail to address it—may eventually lead to infidelity, breakups, and divorce. (For the latest research on sexual boredom, check out "Bored in the Bedroom?" on page 40.)

That's why it's so important to talk about your differences, reach an understanding, and learn how to compromise in a way that helps both of you step outside your usual roles without sacrificing excitement *or* safety. Fortunately, that's not as tough as you'd imagine. Even better, it's entirely possible for both individuals and couples to transform themselves from comfort creatures to thrill seekers if they wish. The key? It's all about communication.

LISA'S STORY: THE PERFECT COMBINATION

After almost twenty years together, my husband, Harry, and I pretty much know each other inside and out. For many long-term couples, two decades is nothing, but in Hollywood, where people tend to change spouses the way starlets change Manolo Blahniks, we're practically old-timers. If you're in a long-term relationship, you know that so much togetherness can be both comforting and challenging. Harry and I are no different: I love that he makes me feel safe and adored, but, like a lot of women, I've gone through periods where I just didn't feel sexy anymore. But, as we've discovered, monogamy doesn't have to equal boring! Our sex life now is hotter than ever, and the reason has a lot to do with our willingness to try new things.

Maybe that means we're thrill seekers, but I like to think we're the perfect combination of both libido types. I have to admit, though, that things weren't always so perfect. When I first met Harry, I wasn't nearly as sexually adventurous as I am now. I wouldn't even call my old self a comfort creature—I just wasn't really into sex, period. My previous two relationships had kind of made me an emotional mess. I had been with the first guy for eight and a half years and felt more like his sister than his lover—sex was never a big part of the equation. My second long-term relationship was no better: He was emotionally unavailable, somewhat sadistic, and sexually confused. Needless to say, I wasn't exactly a risk taker, sexually or otherwise!

Harry was also gun-shy about relationships, having just come out of a dysfunctional relationship of his own. But we took a chance on love—and each other—and have been best friends and soul mates ever since. Having such a caring partner really helped me open up: I credit Harry with what I consider my first sexual awakening, back when we first started dating. And he helped me get my mojo back a second time, after the birth of our two daughters (more about that later on!).

In both cases, we found that while we definitely have a bit of a comfort creature in us—after twenty years, how can you not?—we're also open to pushing boundaries. That didn't used to come naturally to me, though: I may sometimes play a bombshell on screen, but in real life, it took a lot of encouragement and patience from Harry and a big leap of faith on my part to feel as free and relaxed in bed as I do these days. I've learned that trying new things can be scary, but it can also be exhilarating. Thankfully, we trust each other enough that we're able to be "game" and seek out those fun thrills as a couple. I really believe that good sex creates an intimate bond between two people like nothing else, and that helps us feel comfortable getting a little more daring, whether that means doing some sexy role-playing or watching porn together.

HOW ADVENTUROUS ARE YOU?

Lisa and Harry aren't the only couple that enjoys experimenting in the bedroom. Results of a new survey from Good in Bed suggest that men and women of all ages in committed relationships are getting pretty adventurous behind closed doors—and sometimes, out in the open! If you and your partner are looking for ways to break out of your mold and jazz up your usual routine, take some inspiration from these adventuresome respondents. Yeah, yeah, we know what our mothers would say: "Would you jump off a bridge just because your friends did?" Well, no . . . but there's something to be said for reviewing your options. Who knows? You might just find some ideas for spicing up your own sex life.

Good in Bed asked visitors to its website to spill some of their deepest sexual secrets, specifically, what types of risks they had taken in the bedroom. The results? These three thousand men and women—average folks just like you—are surprisingly willing to experience new things in bed. Even better, many of them report that their new adventures increase their sexual satisfaction. Here, the top twelve thrills from the survey:

- Keeping the lights on during sex (89 percent)

- Having sex in your home but outside the bedroom (84 percent)

- Using lubricants during sex (81 percent)

- Talking dirty in bed (65 percent)

- Using a sex toy (such as a vibrator) with a partner (63 percent)

- Wearing sexy lingerie or underwear (61 percent)

- Engaging in voyeuristic behavior, such as watching your partner masturbate or shower (60 percent)

- Having sex with a chance of being seen or overheard (such as at a friend's or family member's home) (57 percent)

- Engaging in exhibitionist behavior, such as masturbating for a partner (52 percent)

- Sharing fantasies verbally (52 percent)

- Watching porn together (50 percent)

- Spanking during sex (48 percent)

Also on the list but ranking a bit lower: reading erotica together, role-playing, engaging in anal sex, indulging in fetishes, and having threesomes. Of course, some of the activities in the top twelve are more adventurous than others—good news for comfort creatures who want to expand their horizons without taking big sexual risks.

YOU MIGHT BE A THRILL SEEKER IF . . .

- You own handcuffs, a nurse's uniform, and stripper shoes—but you're actually an accountant.

- You never buy a piece of furniture without considering how many ways you can have sex on it.

- Acrobatics, riding crops, and a trapeze? Nah, not the circus, just your bedroom.

- You and your partner have christened every room in your house—and every dark alley in your neighborhood.

- The best sex is like an all-you-can eat buffet: tons of variety and unlimited servings!

YOU MIGHT BE A COMFORT CREATURE IF . . .

- Your idea of a hot new bedroom accessory is sheets with a higher thread count.

- You love it when a guy flips your switch—as long as it has a dimmer.

- For you, public sex means doing it in front of a mirror.

- You prefer hot fudge sauce on a sundae, not your partner.

- The best sex is like a big bowl of mac 'n' cheese: It may not be very exotic, but you'd happily indulge again and again.

5

MEETING IN
THE MIDDLE

a couple comprised of two comfort creatures or two thrill seekers definitely has it easier when it comes to sex. But what about the rest of us? Different libido types are not always a problem: Maybe you've already figured out how to compromise in bed, or you believe you're compatible despite your differences. Can you will yourself to be compatible? It may be possible, according to Kristen Mark, a sexuality researcher at Indiana University. She and her colleagues have found that a couple's *perception* of sexual compatibility is much more important to their relationship satisfaction than compatibility of specific turn-ons and turnoffs. For example, if you believe that you and your partner are really sexually compatible—even if your guy likes having sex in bright public places and you prefer sex in dimly lit private spaces—you'll feel just as satisfied with your relationship as people who truly *do* have matching libido types.

If the disparity bothers you, though, and you haven't communicated this to each other, you may find yourselves dealing with a whole lot of hurt feelings and misunderstanding. We really can't stress this enough: You've got to talk with your partner about your concerns. We know, we know—easier said than done. (Trust us, even as sexually open people in long marriages, we both still cringe a bit at the idea of having The Talk with our spouses.) But think about it this way: You're willing to *have* sex with this guy; you should be able to *talk about* sex with him. If you just can't go there, you're not doing yourselves any favors. In fact, being too introverted and fearful of change may be a detriment to your relationship, according to two studies published in the May 2010 issue of *Personality and Social Psychology Bulletin*. Researchers found that shy people have more marital strife than their less-timid peers, possibly because they feel less confident dealing with the inevitable problems that accompany long-term relationships.

BORED IN THE BEDROOM?

Think you're the only one in the sexual doldrums? Think again. A 2011 survey by Good in Bed (conducted with the support of K-Y Brand) found that a whopping *50 percent* of its three thousand respondents said they were either bored in bed or on the brink of boredom. That's a lot of restless nights! Sexual incompatibility and boredom can often go hand in hand because mismatched libidos can mean that at least one partner isn't getting his or her needs met. Other findings from the Good in Bed survey:

- 25 percent of people reported being bored in their relationship, with another 25 percent claiming to be on the brink of boredom.

- The top three sources of boredom were frequency of sex with partner and lack thereof (almost 44 percent), lack of communication with partner (39 percent), and lack of relationship happiness (almost 35 percent).

- 25 percent of people reported having engaged in infidelity due to boredom in their relationship.

Yikes! Numbers like that are enough to make you give up on relationships altogether. But don't despair. There's good news, too: The majority of the respondents (58 percent) were entirely interested in trying something new in the bedroom, with an additional 26 percent mostly or somewhat interested in trying something new. That's a good reason to start seeking some thrills with your partner!

So have a chat about your libidos, no matter how uncomfortable it makes you. (Tip: Don't have the conversation in bed, and definitely don't have it before or during sex.) Not sure of your libido type? Grab your partner and a pen and take this quiz together. Cuddle up on the couch and indulge in a glass of wine or a few pieces of chocolate (remember what chocolate does for your brain's feel-good reward centers!) to turn it into a fun, sexy project rather than an interrogation.

QUIZ: WHAT'S YOUR SEXUAL PERSONALITY?

Not sure if you're a comfort creature, a thrill seeker, or somewhere in between? Take our quiz with your partner to find out.

1) What's more likely to be on or in your bedside table?

A. A photo of your partner, maybe some condoms, and if you're lucky a bottle of lube and a vibrator for your own use.

B. Bedside table? You need a toy chest, and it's filled with a variety of condoms and lube, a pair of handcuffs, and a couple of different vibrators to use with your partner.

2) What's in your wardrobe?

A. A few pieces of tasteful lingerie.

B. Crotchless panties, a French maid's costume, leather chaps, and a whip.

3) What's your favorite place to have sex?

A. Your bedroom.

B. Your kitchen counter, dining room table, the backseat of your car, the beach—anywhere *but* your bed.

4) How often do your fantasies focus on sexual taboos (such as bondage, voyeurism, threesomes, etc.)?

   A. Rarely or never.

   B. Often or all the time.

5) How do you feel about having sex with more than one person at a time?

   A. All I need is my man—no guest stars necessary.

   B. I have fantasized about or had multiple partners at one time—the more, the merrier. And I'm not averse to turning fantasy into reality.

6) Your favorite online video site is:

   A. YouTube

   B. Xtube

7) Whipped cream, chocolate sauce, and cherries . . .

   A. Are the perfect toppings for an ice cream sundae.

   B. Are the perfect toppings for my partner's body.

8) Sex by candlelight is . . .

   A. Romantic and flattering.

   B. A perfect opportunity to play with hot wax.

9) When it comes to sexual positions, you enjoy:

   A. One or more of the old standbys—missionary, woman on top, side by side, or doggy-style.

   B. Working your way through the *Kama Sutra,* one acrobatic position at a time.

10) The perfect date with your partner would end with . . .

    A. Satisfying sex, spooning in bed, and a good night's sleep.

    B. One of you in restraints and a blindfold.

You're finished! Now tally up your A's and B's to find out your libido type.

If you chose mostly A's, you're a *comfort creature*. You enjoy good sex, but you don't require too many extra bells and whistles in bed. Your partner, a few favorite positions, and a dimmer switch are all you need to feel satisfied.

If you chose mostly B's, you're a *thrill seeker*. For you, sex is all about upping the ante with crazy adventures. Toys, props, costumes, and porn are all part of the riskiness you crave.

Now share your answers with your partner to see if you're compatible, or whether it's time to compromise.

THE SEXY ART OF COMPROMISE

Once you've discovered and acknowledged your different libido types, it's time to get busy—literally. For many people, though, it's a lot easier to think about finding sexual common ground than to actually do so. Comfort creatures may feel hesitant to try new things, while thrill seekers may be concerned that compromise will cramp their style. Not to worry: Meeting in the middle sexually is less about giving up yourself than about giving *of* yourself. Simply put, you and your partner just need to embrace the exercises in this chapter with an open mind and an open heart. Remember, you're in this together. Just as you can ignore sexual incompatibility—and allow it to potentially damage your relationship—you can work as a team to take those first steamy steps toward a hotter, more satisfying sex life.

Give Yourself Permission

Today, the Internet and twenty-four-hour cable news channels mean we've got round-the-clock exposure to any number of sex scandals. From Tiger Woods and Jesse James, to John Edwards and Anthony Weiner, there's no shortage of bad boys these days. While it makes great fodder for late-night comedians, such misconduct may make some women even less open to trying new things sexually. As Lisa says, "All that bad male behavior can be an immediate turnoff for a lot of us—we associate sexual risks with perverts rather than with committed relationships. We're more likely to roll our eyes and say 'Eww, what a jerk!' than to experiment with things like sexting or watching porn with our partners."

Instead, we encourage you to reclaim those thrills and make them your own. Are we suggesting that you "tweet" nude pics of yourself to your Twitter followers? No way! But why not text a saucy photo or message to your man, for his eyes only? Or shop together for a sexy movie? There's no reason why you and your partner shouldn't indulge in "risks" like these within your relationship. So give yourself permission to cut loose—we're pretty sure your guy will thank you. For more ideas, see "Good Idea: Sexy Thrills" on page 48.

Get Zen About Sex

There's no doubt about it: Life can be stressful. Whether you're worried about the economy, your job, your kids (or lack thereof), or just those dirty dishes in the sink, there's a seemingly endless list of woes that can drop sex to dead last on your to-do list. Later, we're going to talk a lot more about how stress can affect your sex life (and his!), and you'll learn easy tricks to tune out so you can turn on. For now, just remember that in general, women really need to feel relaxed to be able to let go and enjoy sex—particularly if that sex involves trying new things. Whether it means asking for help around the house, practicing stress management techniques, or making special sex "dates" with your partner, do what you can to let yourself live in the (sexy) moment. Although research suggests that a man's ability to get turned on is less dictated by outside concerns, stress can certainly affect a man's mojo, too. These same approaches can help your guy unwind and get out of his sexual shell as well.

Think Dirty

One of the easiest ways for comfort creatures to push their boundaries is to think—and talk—about what turns them on. If you're both content with your sexual relationship, no problem: Maybe you're already incorporating a favorite fantasy into sex and you're perfectly pleased with the results. But if one of you is a confirmed comfort creature while the other craves more excitement, it may be time to spice things up. The thing that makes fantasies so great is that they're just that: fantasies. There's no rule that dictates that you must act out your fantasy (although it can be great if you do). In his work with couples, Ian has found that the very act of sharing a fantasy with your partner can trigger some pretty hot sex that satisfies both libido types.

Start by determining what turns you on. We all have something that really rocks our boat, even if we've never consciously explored it. Get a journal and a pen and get comfortable, then follow the exercise ("Try This: What Turns You On?") on page 46 to delve deeper into your fantasies. Then it's time to share those thoughts with your partner. The ideal time to discuss your erotic thoughts is during foreplay, because when your guy is aroused, the flood of chemicals to his brain will lower his inhibitions. If you're not sure how to bring up the subject, tell him that you had a sexy dream about him. When he asks for more details (trust us, he'll want to know), whisper some sexy snippets in his ear.

Want to know *his* fantasies? You can try to get him talking by asking if it turns him on, too, or what he would do in that situation. If he's still tongue-tied, you might be able to draw him into a conversation with some simple yes-or-no questions, such as "Would you want to have sex with me and another woman?" or "Would you like me to blindfold you?" Then, when he responds, ask him to elaborate. Hopefully, by you being up-front about your desires, he'll be more

try this: WHAT TURNS YOU ON?

In the romantic comedy *When Harry Met Sally,* Meg Ryan's character shares her deepest, hottest fantasy with Billy Crystal's Harry: A faceless stranger rips her clothes off. *That's it?* Harry wonders incredulously. "Sometimes I vary it a little," she replies. "I change what I'm wearing." The joke may humorously highlight the differences between men and women, but it also proves our point: Any fantasy is a good fantasy if it turns you on!

Everybody has fantasies, whether they stem from a memorable sexual experience, a scene in a movie or book, or just your imagination. In this exercise, you're going to uncover what makes *you* hot. Grab a journal and pen and write down your answers to the following questions. Don't second-guess or judge yourself—just jot down whatever you're thinking. Once you're done, brainstorm ways you might incorporate these fictions into reality if you wish. Remember, just sharing your thoughts with your partner can be a huge turn-on for both of you.

- What is your favorite or most recurring sexual fantasy?

- Which elements of the fantasy particularly arouse you—which ones do you replay over and over in your mind?

- Have you ever shared this fantasy with your partner?

- Do you use this fantasy to get turned on during or before having sex with your partner or masturbating?

- How has this fantasy changed over time?

- Why do you think it's so powerful for you?

- Would you like to play out your fantasy in reality? If so, how would you raise the subject comfortably with your partner?

open about his, too. Whether you decide to act out your fantasies is up to the two of you, but simply sharing them can help both of you shake things up a bit.

Seduce Him

Trying to step outside your comfort zone with a thrill-seeking partner? Or maybe your guy is less experimental but you'd like him to join you in a walk on the wild side? Either way, a little role-playing can help ease comfort creatures into riskier fun while keeping thrill seekers from getting bored—all within the safety of your relationship. According to a recent study at the University of British Columbia, all you need is your hot selves, plus a few key props and a vivid imagination. Researchers there found that longtime couples were best able to rekindle romance by pretending they were strangers on a first date. So play around with wigs and different outfits, assume an alias, and meet your partner at a local restaurant or bar for a rendezvous. Call on your man to deliver a pizza, fix the cable, or otherwise show up at your door with a different persona. Sounds cheesy, but it works. You get variety and safety—and a hot new way to compromise.

Don't Give up on Intimacy

Sometimes, no matter how hard you both try, you're going to hit some roadblocks. Maybe you feel as if you've pushed your willingness to take risks to its limits, or perhaps your partner's sex drive is in a lull. If you find yourselves at odds—and on opposite sides of the bed—keep in mind that your differences may be temporary. Sex can be more important in a relationship at certain times, and other times it fades into the background because of other priorities or responsibilities, or because you feel disconnected. Sexual desire ebbs and flows naturally over the course of a relationship—and over the course of your life.

One solution is to embrace your libido and desire differences and find a type and frequency that works for both of you. If you want more or racier sex

good idea: SEXY THRILLS

Looking for fun ways to inject a little risk into your sex life? Even confirmed comfort creatures can feel at ease with these tips.

a) Leave the lights on during sex.

b) Buy a new brand of lubricant (flavored varieties are fun, too) and try it out.

c) Send your partner a sexy e-mail or voice mail message describing a fantasy or your plans with him for the evening (be sure to use his personal, not company, account!).

d) "Sext" a spicy message or photo to his cell phone.

e) Engage in a little "Skype sex" to fan the flames if one of you is out of town—or as a fun form of foreplay, even if he's in the next room.

f) Rent a sexy movie and act out what you see on screen.

g) Wear a piece of sexy lingerie in bed.

h) Masturbate for your partner or ask him to do the same for you.

i) Talk dirty in bed.

j) Think about your favorite fantasies and brainstorm how you can reenact them by playing with costumes, props, and sex toys.

k) Agree to have sex in any room in your house other than your bedroom. Up the ante by moving to your car or making out in a semipublic place like a dark theater or alley (don't get caught!).

than your partner, consider what you really want. Is your goal to have more orgasms more often? If so, masturbate some of the time and incorporate fantasies, erotica, or porn into those solo sex sessions. If it's simply physical intimacy with your partner you crave, perhaps you can share a bath or a massage with him—without the expectation of sex. Make sure to kiss and hug each other just for the sake of kissing and hugging, without trying to have sex. Once you stop making every gesture of affection a proposition for sex, you may find that your guy starts initiating more often.

If you're the one who wants less sex or fewer thrills, be clear about what you're saying no to, because your partner is apt to feel unattractive or rejected. Explain that you don't want to have sex because you're tired, or having a rough week, or upset today, or that you just don't have the same level of desire as him. (Make it clear that low desire is your issue, not a reaction to him.) Help him understand, then try to say yes some of the times you want to say no, to meet in the middle. You just may find that as you kiss, hug, and take things further, you begin to get in the mood.

part three

·

sexual
CONFIDENCE

We'll spend a lot of time in this book talking about your sex life with your partner and the importance of exuding confidence in bed. The fact is, though, that a state of boldness and self-assurance isn't always so easy to attain. Perhaps that's because so many women place the responsibility for that feeling squarely on the shoulders of their partner: According to a survey by *Men's Health* magazine, 75 percent of women cite their husbands or boyfriends as the main source of their sexual confidence.

While we're all for partners that make you feel like the vixen we know you are, a man's encouragement and approval shouldn't be the *only* basis for a woman's self-esteem. Put it this way: If you know you're kicking butt at the office, do you really need a pat on the head from a male colleague to know you're doing a great job? The same should hold true in all facets of your life, including the bedroom. True belief in yourself comes from within, and its effects will be obvious to anyone who sees your glowing face and confident stride.

Of course, getting to that place of self-assurance can take time, effort, and the willingness to be vulnerable. Sexually speaking, that means becoming comfortable with your body, identifying and overcoming issues that may sap your mojo, and giving yourself permission to relax, let go, and enjoy yourself. That's what this section of *The Big, Fun, Sexy Sex Book* is all about.

LISA'S STORY:
JOURNEY TO SELF-CONFIDENCE

A lot of people assume that because I'm an actress I've always been super-confident, both in and out of bed. They're wrong. The truth is, I grew up feeling very self-conscious: I was an only child, my parents moved when I was seven (which made it difficult to make new friends), and my "exotic" looks made me stand out. Not only was I the new kid at school, but I looked different, too. Children can be cruel, and I was picked on and made fun of for much of my childhood.

Sure, Lisa, you're saying. But then you grew up and became a famous actress, married the "Sexiest Man Alive," and posed for *Playboy*. You must have felt confident by then. Um, not exactly. Acting, like a lot of other professions, involves a lot of rejection. Some of it is based on talent and whether you're right for a certain role, but much of it is based on appearance: You're too tall, too short, too young, too old, too exotic, or not exotic enough. And before I met Harry, I dated a man on whom I totally depended for my self-esteem—and who was able to tear me down with just a few words or a look. After much soul-searching (and therapy), I realized that I'd hit rock bottom in the confidence department. It was time to stop looking to everyone else to build me up, and start looking within myself.

More than twenty years later, I finally feel good—no, great—about myself. It's taken a lot of hard work to get here: Therapy, spiritual practices such as yoga, and books that teach how to live in the moment, such as those by Eckhart Tolle, have been invaluable to me in this journey. I've realized that not everyone is always going to like me, but now I see negative experiences as opportunities—those teasing kids, my unsupportive boyfriend, the often-harsh media have all taught me hard but valuable lessons and have only made me stronger. In the end, true belief in yourself is what really matters. And what's sexier than that?

6

GETTING TO
KNOW YOU

t here is so much darkness and secrecy surrounding them," writes Eve Ensler
in her play *The Vagina Monologues*. "Like the Bermuda Triangle, no one
ever reports back from there." A woman's genitals have long seemed like the
most mysterious of body parts, intimidating to some in their complexity. In fact,
they're not that complicated at all, just mostly hidden from plain sight. But it
doesn't help that unless she's a gynecologist, the average heterosexual woman
has few opportunities to view very many vaginas other than her own. Even if
you grew up reading Judy Blume novels and perusing *Our Bodies, Ourselves,* the
pictures of female genitals you're exposed to now are probably limited to what
you see in men's magazines, porn, and the occasional celebrity wardrobe mal-
function. And that can add to those feelings of concern about whether you're
"normal" down there, especially since a lot of what we see in print has been
airbrushed into someone else's idea of perfection.

That's why it's so important to familiarize yourself with your own reproductive anatomy. If you haven't already done so, grab a hand mirror and hit a well-
lit (and private) room for a little exploration and discovery. Let's get acquainted,
shall we?

BASIC FEMALE ANATOMY

Before we get started, let's get something straight: "Vagina" is not the proper word for everything between your legs. It's kind of funny, actually: Men and women alike tend to be uncomfortable even saying the word *vagina*—yet they use it to describe the whole female genital area. In fact, there are myriad aspects to a woman's genitals:

VULVA. *This* is actually the collective name for all of a woman's external genitalia, except for the urethra, which isn't technically part of the reproductive system, despite its location.

LABIA MAJORA. These are the soft, stretchy lips on the outside of the vulva. Bikini waxes not withstanding, they're usually covered with hair on one side.

LABIA MINORA. These are the delicate, sensitive lips inside the vulva. They're typically some shade of pink (regardless of your ethnicity) and darken and swell when you're aroused.

LABIAL COMMISSURE. On your mouth, the commissures are the corners where your lips meet. You've got two commissures on your vulva, too: one at the top and one at the bottom where the labia meet.

CLITORIS. For many women, this is the pleasure center during sex. And no wonder: The clitoris has more nerve fibers—eight thousand of them—than any other part of the human body and interacts with the fifteen thousand nerve fibers that service the entire pelvic area. Plus, despite its moniker as a "love button," the clitoris is much larger than it appears. Like the penis, it has three components—a head, a shaft, and a base—with some visible parts on the surface of the vulva and other unseen parts inside the vaginal area. Some researchers have identified a whopping eighteen structures as part of the clitoris. And recent research even suggests the G-spot may actually just be the back-end roots of the clitoris.

VAGINA. Also known as the birth canal, the average vagina is just three inches long when not aroused. It's made of delicate tissue that "sweats," or lubricates, when you're turned on. Even though a lot of people may equate the vagina with the penis in terms of sexuality and pleasure, only the outer third of it is particularly sensitive. A better comparison is the penis and the clitoris.

PERINEUM. This is the area between the bottom of the vaginal opening and the anus.

ANUS. The anus is a delicate ring of muscle that is densely packed with nerve endings and extremely responsive to light touch and deep pressure.

Just as a man's body changes when he's aroused, so does a woman's. When you're turned on, blood flow to the genitals increases, which helps trigger the production of vaginal lubrication and causes swelling in the clitoris, labia minora, labia majora, and vagina. As your arousal continues, the labia minora and majora may swell and their natural color may deepen. The vagina expands and lengthens, too, as the uterus is pulled upward into the body, changing the position of the cervix. The vaginal opening tightens and the clitoris retracts underneath the clitoral hood, protecting the nerve-rich clitoris from direct stimulation, which can be uncomfortable for some women. You may also notice feelings of tingling, throbbing, and fullness throughout your pelvic area.

POP QUIZ

According to iVillage.com, what percentage of married women fantasize about sex with someone who is not their spouse?

(A) 12 percent   **(B)** 62 percent   **(C)** 75 percent   **(D)** 99 percent

Correct Answer: (B) 62 percent. Interestingly, women do tend to fantasize during sex more than men. Researchers believe that women need to relax and mentally disconnect during sex in order to reach orgasm. Fantasy helps facilitate that process of mental deactivation. And just because a woman is fantasizing about someone else doesn't mean she's interested in actually having sex with that person. Fantasies are fantasies for a reason—because they're not real. Instead of feeling threatened, why not reenact the fantasy and get some wild sex out of it?

WHAT'S UP "DOWN THERE"?

Vulvas are kind of like snowflakes (and penises, for that matter): Each one is unique. You'd never know it, though, from the media's portrayal of female genitals. Pornography in particular has created an unrealistic standard of small, perfectly symmetrical labia and bare vulvas. But that perfection can come at a price: If a porn star's genitals don't fit the mold of what's considered attractive, she may even go under the knife to make them more in line with that industry's standard of beauty. That surgery, known as labiaplasty, trims the size of the labia minora and is on the rise among non-porn stars as well. The problem? The labia are rich with nerve endings—and surgically altering them could decrease your sexual pleasure or even make intercourse painful. Yikes!

In truth, very few women have naturally porn-standardized genitals. And while a small number of men may make disparaging jokes to each other about the size and shape of vulvas—some guys *are* jerks, after all—the majority of men are pretty happy just to be near one, especially if it belongs to a woman they're really into. So learn to accept and embrace your differences. We think confidence about your body is the best aphrodisiac, and research backs us up: According to a study published in the January 2011 issue of the *Journal of Sexual Medicine,* a positive genital self-image is significantly related to good female sexual function. Here are some more facts about what goes on "down there":

SIZE, SHAPE, AND SYMMETRY. The appearance of the labia minora, or inner lips, varies from woman to woman, and almost all iterations are normal. They can be gently curved, scalloped, or wavy; barely noticeable or long enough to extend past the labia majora (outer lips); and, like your breasts and feet, one side may be larger than the other. There may even be some benefit to having longer labia minora: They can increase friction during intercourse, which can in turn increase pleasure for both you and your partner.

BOUNCING BACK. When you think about it, the vagina is fairly amazing. It can expand to accommodate intercourse and childbirth and yet contract to its original size afterward. Many women (and men) believe that too much sex, a large partner, or use of certain sex toys will permanently make the vagina larger. These concerns have more to do with feelings of male size insecurity, guilt, shame, or anxiety about sex than they do with the physical facts. Many women believe too much sex will "mark" their bodies in some way, or are pestered about vaginal tightness by a partner who worries he doesn't match up to a former partner. Can you imagine how ridiculous it would sound if a man thought his penis would shrink as he had more sex?

In fact, the vagina is an incredibly elastic organ that is designed to accommodate different sizes and return to its baseline shape afterward. The vagina is a potential space, meaning that it can grow in size to accommodate a penis or a baby, then contract afterward. No matter how much sex a woman has, her vagina will not permanently change in size in any substantial way. Even women who have had a partner with a large penis or used large sex toys will find their vagina adapts to future sexual activity. If you're still worried about a loss of tightness, you can do Kegel exercises to strengthen the muscles surrounding the vagina (see "A Different Kind of Workout" on page 149).

try this: TURN ON . . . THE LIGHTS!

When you're uncomfortable with your body, it's tempting to hide in the dark or under the covers during sex. But here's one situation where you really should fake it till you make it. Even if you're seriously self-conscious, the simple act of pretending that you're brimming with boldness about your body can make you seem hotter to your partner—and yourself: That rush of accomplishment you feel when you face your fears can be a big turn-on for both of you.

NATURALLY CLEAN. Vaginal discharge is one of those things most women just don't want to talk about. Changes in vaginal discharge, however, can teach a woman about her body and alert her when something might be wrong. The vagina produces secretions to prevent it from becoming dry, as well as to maintain a healthy pH balance to fight off infection. Most women find that discharge changes over the course of a menstrual cycle and as a result of aging. Many medications, overall health, and dietary and lifestyle choices also can affect a woman's discharge. In general, women in their childbearing years will find that discharge is lightest during and just after a period, and creamier, more abundant, or slippery as she approaches ovulation.

Keeping track of daily discharge can help you learn what's normal for your body. Pay attention to sensations of wetness and the appearance of discharge in underwear. Discharge that is excessive, smells different, or changes color, especially if accompanied by itching or burning, should be checked out by a health-care provider. Most vaginal infections are easily treated but can lead to complications if left untreated. And remember, since the vagina is self-cleaning, douching interferes with the natural balance and can actually increase your risk of infection and your production of discharge.

A HAIRY SITUATION

Just glance at a photo of a nude woman from a few decades ago and you'll remember that, yes, natural pubic hair was once in style. These days, though, the trend has been to remove most or all of the hair "down there." And although it's mainly a female thing, a number of guys are getting in on the act, too, "manscaping" the hair around the penis and even the testicles (ouch!). As is often the case, we have pornography to thank for this fad: Niche films aside, find us a current porn star who's got more than the tiniest landing strip of hair.

Actually, there's no single standard of grooming and no reason, hygienically speaking, to remove pubic hair. Like the hair on our heads, how and if you style it should be a matter of personal choice. Indeed, a study of more than 2,450 women, published in the October 2010 issue of the *Journal of Sexual Medicine*, found a diverse range of pubic hair grooming practices. A 2009 study in the same journal suggested that such grooming can be an important part of a woman's sexual expression.

That said, shaving, trimming, depilatory, waxing, and laser treatment can provide a range of possibilities for those who wish to go a little or a lot more bare. And you may find that experimenting with different styles may spice things up between you and your partner, increase sensitivity in the genitals, and make them more accessible for oral sex. From au natural, to a simple trim, to the "landing strip" (a thin vertical rectangle), to the full Brazilian (completely bare), you've got a lot of options. Do what feels right, and fun, for you.

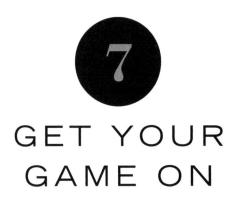

GET YOUR
GAME ON

even if you're comfortable with your sexual anatomy, you still may not feel exactly bold in bed. Sure, some of us are born confident. But for many people, self-esteem is something that doesn't come naturally. This can be a particular challenge for women, who tend to be told from a young age that they should stifle their sexuality: *Don't move your hips like that! A lady always crosses her legs. Good girls don't act like that* . . . and on and on. These lessons might be fine for kids, but they can still mess with your confidence when you're an adult. The truth is, good girls (or, more accurately, women) do—and enjoy—a lot of things, and there's nothing wrong with that. But how do you go from skittish to sexually bold? It's all about your attitude.

LISA'S STORY: HOW TO BE GAME

I talk a lot in this book about "being game" in bed. That doesn't mean that I do whatever a man tells me, but it does mean that I'm up for anything—or at least thinking about anything—in my relationship with my husband. To me, being game is being bold, fearless, and open to trying something new sexually, as long as it's consensual.

Of course, being game isn't familiar to most of us—and it didn't used to come naturally to me, either. As an actress, I've always been pretty skilled at pretending to be confident. But the real thing didn't come to me until 2006.

That was the year that I joined the cast of *Dancing with the Stars,* and it's not an understatement to say that the experience changed my life. I've written about *DWTS* before, in my book *Rinnavation,* but I just can't say enough about what an impact it had on me. I'd been invited to join the first season of the show and regretted turning it down, so I jumped at the chance to join the second season and dance with my professional partner, Louis Van Amstel.

Boy, was I in for a surprise! Dance—and exercise in general—has long been an important part of my life. I took and taught Jazzercise for years, and by 2006 I'd also tried Tae Bo, rock-and-roll yoga, and of course, Sheila Kelley's fabulous S Factor pole-dancing classes. But nothing had prepared me for the grueling all-day practice sessions—or the thrill of dancing in front of a live studio and television audience. It was both harder and more rewarding than anything I'd done in my life. Yes, it changed my body for the better (I lost ten pounds and three inches from my waist). But the biggest effects were emotional. I felt like years of pent-up emotions were just flowing from me with the tears I cried during most rehearsals: I was scared, frustrated, and exhilarated, all at the same time.

Right about now, you're probably saying, "That's great, Lisa. But what on earth does *Dancing with the Stars* have to do with my sex life?" It's simple, really. Facing my fears and emotions by trying something new gave me a greater sense of power and confidence than ever before. I totally opened up my mind and my body, and the results carried over from the dance studio to the bedroom.

So when women ask me what they can do to gain sexual confidence, I tell them about *DWTS.* But you don't need to master the rhumba or the fox-trot to benefit—unless, of course, you want to! Just think of something you've always wanted to learn or do but have always been too afraid to try. We all have something. Maybe you love singing alone in the shower or the car, but

lisa says . . . ACT AS IF

Several years ago, I was in Malibu at a birthday luncheon for a good friend of mine. There were about ten women there—including Barbra Streisand, another friend of the birthday girl. It was a gorgeous day, and as we relaxed, ate, and engaged in girl talk, my friend said, "Hey, Lisa! Tell everyone the story about how you got your mojo back." So I launched into the tale I've shared with you here: Lou Paget's sex-tip classes, Sheila Kelley's S Factor, buying sexy costumes and playing dress-up for Harry. As I wrapped up my story, Ms. Streisand, who was seated across from me, leaned over, fascinated. "You mean," she said, "that you make an effort? That is so amazing!"

You wouldn't think that "making an effort" would be so intriguing. But the truth is that many women—many couples—don't. I think a lot of us believe that great sex just happens, or that the man will do all the work in bed, or that guys love sex, so we just have to show up. Not true! We women bear just as much responsibility for our sex lives. Now, I'm certainly not saying that it's our job to keep things sexy and fun. It should be a team approach. But it doesn't hurt to, as Ms. Streisand put it, make an effort.

The challenge, though, is feeling confident enough in bed to make that effort easily. As I discussed earlier, learning how to be game is one way to boost your self-esteem. Another way you can start acting bolder? It's a tip I learned during years of acting classes, and it applies to all parts of life, not just sexuality: Act as if. Over the course of my career, I've had to act as if I were a variety of women, from recovering drug addict Billie Reed in *Days of Our Lives,*

you're too terrified to even attempt karaoke or join your church choir. Take voice lessons. Have you always enjoyed doodling but never thought you were good enough to go further? Try a drawing or painting class. Do you like poetry but are afraid to share your poems with others? Join a writing workshop.

to scheming seductress Taylor McBride in *Melrose Place,* to homicidal showgirl Roxie Hart in Broadway's *Chicago.* These characters were all so different that I had to believe that I was them to truly embody them.

You might not be an actress, but you can—and should—still try this approach. I'm not suggesting that you fake orgasm, of course. But a little make-believe can go a long way. Think about it: We all played pretend as kids, whether we imagined being pretty princesses, or tough policewomen, or president of the United States. We've all been someone who we aren't—and being that character can infuse us with confidence.

Consider most of today's female pop stars. Britney, Christina, Madonna, J. Lo, Lady Gaga . . . they all project sensual, bold stage personas. But I'd be willing to bet that none of these women is quite so over-the-top sexy in real life. They have bad hair days and bad moods and frumpy phases just like the rest of us. So what's different? They're putting on a show. I love that Beyoncé has admitted that she overcame her stage fright by creating a sexy, confident alter ego named Sasha Fierce that allows her to feel comfortable gyrating and shaking her booty in front of millions of people.

Why not invent your own Sasha Fierce—your very own inner diva? We've all been trained to put that girl so deep inside us that she's practically in solitary confinement. It's time to let her out! Give her a name, a back story, a look, a wardrobe, an attitude. You probably won't bring her out to play all the time, but you might want to rely on her when you're suggesting and trying something new in bed or when you need an extra boost of confidence. She can be your little secret, but your guy—and your sex life—will definitely see the rewards.

Now you may not become the next Mariah Carey (or Georgia O'Keeffe, or Maya Angelou, for that matter). That's not the important part. Instead, the goal is to test yourself, to face your fears, and to cultivate confidence. I firmly believe that when you become daring outside of bed, your sex life will follow. So create your own *Dancing with the Stars* moment!

part four

·

LISA'S
"get your sexy back"
PLAN

When you read the words *sexual fitness,* images of crazy acrobatic positions probably come to mind. While we're for all experimentation, we're actually talking about your health. You need to feel good to be in the mood for sex, right? With today's stresses—from work woes, to financial worries, to family troubles—that's not so easy. Maybe you scarf down a fast-food meal on the way home from the office or snack on a candy bar as you shuttle your kids to their next appointment. You stay up late working on a big presentation instead of getting adequate sleep. You veg out on the couch with your remote instead of hitting the gym. Then you wonder why sex seems like a distant memory.

It doesn't have to be that way. A healthy lifestyle can take a little time and a lot of commitment, but it will come naturally once you make it a habit. Here's how:

BE ACTIVE. Whether you're looking to lose weight or gain sexual stamina, a cardiovascular workout should always be a part of your regular exercise regimen. Women who *don't* exercise are more likely to experience arousal issues, because regular aerobic workouts help to keep the blood flowing to your genitals, as well as release feel-good endorphins that contribute to relaxation and sexual arousal. Exercise also plays a major role in generating positive self-esteem—perhaps the most powerful sexual enhancer.

EAT WELL. A poor diet is a major contributor to heart disease, high cholesterol, arterial plaque, and high blood pressure, among other conditions, all of which inhibit blood flow to the genitals and impact both desire and arousal. The more nutrient-dense foods you consume, the more you will be satisfied with fewer calories, and the less you will crave more high-calorie foods.

MANAGE STRESS AND SLEEP. As we've said before, stress can take a major toll on your sex life. Obviously, our sex lives themselves can be a source of stress and anxiety, all of which can create a vicious, destructive cycle. To have a healthy sex life, you have to be in the sort of relationship that supports having a healthy sex life; follow the advice in part 1 of this book. And don't forget about sufficient shut-eye: Sleep is as vital to our physical well-being as food and water, and even a single restless night will find its expression in higher levels of stress and lower levels of arousal. On the other hand, people who are well rested are more able to have better sex.

JUST SAY NO. We all know that tobacco contributes to lung and heart disease, but you may not realize that it can affect sexual health as well. Smoking damages the arteries affecting blood flow to the genitals, leading to a loss of desire and arousal in both men and women. In terms of alcohol consumption, most of us know that having a drink or two before sex may help us relax and ease our inhibitions. But high levels of consumption can also result in sexual dysfunction, including your ability to get or stay aroused. Other chemical substances such as marijuana and cocaine also have known links to low sex drive and sexual dysfunction.

Now that you've gotten a bead on your health, start keeping a daily journal to track how your health affects your sex life. As you go through your day, think about how each daily activity affects your sexual health and whether it fundamentally helps you or hurts you. Once you start to notice the connection between good health and good sex, it will be easier to keep making the right choices for both. Want more guidance? Try Lisa's program, beginning on the next page.

THE SEVEN-DAY PROGRAM

It's simple, really: When you feel healthy, you feel sexy. You have more energy, you're happier, your skin glows, and that all adds up to more confidence, in and out of bed. On the flip side, who wants to be romantic when you're tired, cranky, and bloated? That's why I think taking good care of your body is so important for a vibrant sex life.

This is the program I follow when I need a quick jump start toward good health. Don't be intimidated: It's not a diet—although if you lose a few extra pounds, that's a bonus. Instead, it's a plan that helps you feel lighter, boosts your energy, and lets you feel more in touch with your body. I can't guarantee that you'll have more or better sex, but I truly believe that you'll feel more confident and you just might carry that new self-assuredness into the bedroom.

Give it just seven days and see how you react. Chances are, you'll want to keep it up. (As with any new diet or exercise program, be sure to check with your doctor before starting.)

What to Eat

In general, you should only eat whole, unprocessed foods this week—nothing from a box or a bag. It takes a little planning, but you should be able to pull it off. If I can prepare these meals, then you can, too. (Let's just say I'm never going to be on *Top Chef*!) Shop for the week so you have everything you need, and cut down on prep time by washing and chopping your veggies before you store them in the fridge.

Your basic goal is to eat fewer refined carbohydrates and more lean proteins, which gives you more energy and cuts down on bloat. (Who doesn't want a flatter tummy in bed?) The bad news? You'll have to skip dessert and cut out alcohol for the week. The good news? You can enjoy all the produce you want—fruits and vegetables are great sources of fiber, antioxidants, and other healthful compounds. And be sure to drink plenty of water throughout the day; I add lemon to mine for an extra kick. Here are some meal ideas to get you started. Mix and match the days and meals however you want.

Day One

BREAKFAST
1 cup high-fiber cereal; 1 cup fat-free or soy milk; 1 sliced banana

MIDMORNING SNACK
1 hard-boiled egg; 1 cup baby carrots

LUNCH
1 cup black bean soup; 1 mixed green salad tossed with 1 tablespoon balsamic vinaigrette; 2 high-fiber crackers with 1 slice of low-fat cheese

AFTERNOON SNACK
10 to 15 almonds

DINNER
Asian stir-fry (4 ounces firm cubed tofu, sautéed with bok choy in 2 teaspoons of olive oil and 1 teaspoonful of sesame seeds); ½ cup quinoa; 1 mixed green salad

Day Two

BREAKFAST
Veggie omelet (1 whole egg and 2 egg whites with spinach, tomatoes, and mushrooms); 1 slice whole wheat toast; 1 cup fat-free milk or soy milk

MIDMORNING SNACK

6 carrot or jicama sticks; 2 tablespoons of guacamole

LUNCH

Asian chicken salad (4 ounces of grilled boneless, skinless chicken breast, cucumbers, water chestnuts, scallions, peanuts, and 2 teaspoons each of sesame oil and brown rice vinegar)

AFTERNOON SNACK

1 handful of blueberries and 1 cup vanilla soy milk

DINNER

Turkey burger and 1 slice reduced-fat cheese on a whole wheat bun; 1 handful veggie chips; 1 mixed green salad

Day Three

BREAKFAST

1 cup Greek or nonfat yogurt topped with 1 tablespoon of slivered almonds, 1 teaspoon of wheat germ, and 1 cup of diced mango or berries

MIDMORNING SNACK

10 to 15 almonds and raisins

LUNCH

1 veggie burger with ½ sliced avocado on a whole wheat English muffin, topped with salsa

AFTERNOON SNACK

1 small apple, sliced, and 2 teaspoons nut butter

DINNER

Poached halibut (4 ounces) with lemon, salt and pepper, and olive oil; steamed carrots; 1 mixed green salad

Day Four

BREAKFAST

Egg-white wrap (3 egg whites, scrambled; 1 slice reduced-fat cheese; whole wheat tortilla); 1 nonfat latte

MIDMORNING SNACK

½ cup nonfat cottage cheese with ½ cup cubed pineapple

LUNCH

Open-faced veggie sandwich (grilled zucchini, eggplant, roasted peppers, and artichoke hearts on 1 slice Ezekiel or whole wheat bread, topped with 1 slice part-skim mozzarella cheese and sprouts)

AFTERNOON SNACK

¾ cup Greek yogurt with 3 teaspoons wheat germ

DINNER

Grilled boneless, skinless chicken breast (4 ounces); arugula salad with olive oil and lemon juice dressing; kale chips (top torn pieces of kale with 2 teaspoons of olive oil and sea salt and roast until crispy)

Day Five

BREAKFAST

1 packet organic sugar-free instant oatmeal with 1 teaspoon coconut oil, 1 teaspoon ground flaxseed, and stevia to taste; 1 cup nonfat or soy milk

MIDMORNING SNACK

½ cup steamed edamame (soybeans)

LUNCH

Pasta salad (1/2 cup whole wheat cooked pasta, steamed broccoli, 2 teaspoons Parmesan cheese tossed with ½ cup marinara sauce and topped with 4 ounces chopped cooked chicken, shrimp, or steak [optional])

AFTERNOON SNACK

1 handful of trail mix

DINNER

Grilled steak (4 ounces); steamed broccoli with lemon; spinach salad with 1 ounce goat cheese and 1 ounce slivered almonds

LISA'S DAILY GREEN DRINK

I rarely start my day without this nutrient-packed beverage. It looks a little strange (bright green), but it tastes yummy, feels filling, and keeps my energy up all day long. Just wash and chop the following produce. No need to measure—just use what looks right to you: kale, spinach, cucumber, parsley, celery, apple juice, and a squeeze of lemon. (I always buy organic when possible.) Throw it all into a blender or juicer and process until it's the consistency of a smoothie. Enjoy!

Day Six

BREAKFAST

Egg sandwich (2 scrambled egg whites, diced tomatoes, and sprinkle of reduced-fat cheese on 2 slices Ezkiel or whole wheat bread)

MIDMORNING SNACK

2 high-fiber crackers topped with 2 teaspoons coconut butter

LUNCH

Chopped chef's salad (romaine lettuce, hard-boiled egg whites, tomatoes, cucumbers, celery; 4 ounces chopped cooked boneless, skinless chicken or turkey breast; and 1 teaspoon balsamic vinaigrette)

AFTERNOON SNACK

100-calorie pack of microwave popcorn

DINNER

1 cup whole wheat pasta with ½ cup marinara sauce, sautéed zucchini, and a sprinkle of Parmesan cheese

Day Seven

BREAKFAST

1 protein shake (1 cup nonfat or soy milk, 1 cup ice, 2 teaspoons nut butter, 1 teaspoon cocoa-flavored protein powder)

MIDMORNING SNACK

15 grapes

LUNCH

Grilled chicken salad (4 ounces grilled boneless, skinless chicken breast, chopped, over romaine lettuce, cherry tomatoes, reduced-fat feta cheese, and 1 teaspoon balsamic vinaigrette)

AFTERNOON SNACK

2 slices of turkey on a whole wheat tortilla wrap with 1 teaspoon guacamole

DINNER

Baked wild salmon (4 ounces); mashed cauliflower; steamed green beans

LISA'S ONE-DAY JUMP START

Feeling sluggish, not sexy? This one-day fast helps me feel lighter, brighter, and more energetic—it's like cleaning a window so I can see more clearly. (You might want to try this fast on a Sunday or other day when you aren't too busy.)

7 A.M.: Start your day with 8 ounces of clean water with a spritz of lemon and pinch of cayenne pepper.

9 A.M., 11 a.m., 1 p.m., and 4 p.m.: Drink sixteen to twenty ounces of my special green drink (see recipe on page 74). At 4 p.m., add a shot of wheatgrass juice (available at health food stores).

7 P.M.: Ease out of the fast with a vegetable smoothie or blended vegetable soup. You could also add a light mixed green salad or steamed veggies.

THROUGHOUT THE DAY: Sip herbal tea if you like.

How to Move

I'm a firm believer in the value of exercise: It improves mood, boosts energy, strengthens muscles, and keeps that all-important blood flowing to the genitals. In short, I'd like you to try to get at least thirty minutes of aerobic activity every day. You don't need to join a gym or take a class—unless you want to, of course. And you don't need to get all thirty minutes at once. There are plenty of fun ways to fit in fitness throughout your day, such as running, walking, taking the stairs, dancing around your living room, chasing after your kids, doing yard work or housework, swimming, cycling, taking a spin or boot-camp-style class . . . the list goes on.

I also recommend practicing some sort of stretching and toning activity two or three times a week if you can manage it. You could lift weights or use a strength-training machine, do Pilates, or try yoga. Again, no gym membership is necessary: Most of us have an exercise DVD lying around the house that we bought with the best of intentions and then forgot about. Dig it out and give it a try! Or check out your cable company's "on demand" fitness menu, search online, or download a smartphone app for other free or inexpensive exercise options. I'm a big fan of yoga because it provides a total-body workout while encouraging relaxation through meditation and an awareness of how your mind and body are connected.

Whatever types of exercise you choose, stay active all week long. It doesn't matter whether you lose weight or start to develop a six-pack—those are great benefits, but they're not our goals here. Combined with my whole-food eating plan, you should start feeling better all the way around: Better confidence, both on the streets and between the sheets, will follow!

LISA'S FAVORITE "SEXERCISES"

(Be sure to check with your doctor before beginning any new physical activity and take it slow—a pulled muscle or sprained ankle won't exactly put you in the mood for sex.)

While any type of physical activity can benefit your overall mental and physical health, there are some types of exercise that I turn to time and again when I want to boost my sex life. In particular, I find that yoga and dancing help unlock my sensuality and increase my sexual desire and arousal.

Now I'm not saying that these "sexercises" will absolutely give you better sex, but in my experience, they can help you feel slimmer, calmer, and more sexual. Some even strengthen and tone the muscles you use most during sex—your pelvic floor muscles—and may even improve your chances of mind-blowing orgasms. Here are some of my favorites.

Yoga

These poses can help increase desire and arousal, tone your muscles, build confidence, improve relaxation, and may even make you more orgasmic. Many of them also open up the hips, where a lot of us hold tension (including sexual tension). Although I've been practicing yoga for years, these poses are easy enough for beginners, too. See if you can fit one or all of them into your daily stretching routine.

Bound Angle

- Sit with your legs straight in front of you. If your hamstrings or hips are especially tight, sit on a folded towel or blanket.

- As you exhale, pull your knees toward your pelvis and then let your knees fall open to either side of you.

- Press the soles of your feet together and pull them as close to your pelvis as possible. Grasp the big toe of each foot with your first and second fingers and your thumb. If you can't reach your toes, hold onto your ankles or shins.

- Keep your pelvis in a neutral position and slide your shoulder blades down your back as you lengthen your torso.

- Hold this position for one to five minutes, breathing deeply throughout.

Up Dog

- Lie facedown on the floor, with the tops of your feet on the floor, your palms on the floor by your waist, and your arms bent at a perpendicular angle to the floor.

- As you inhale, press your hands into the floor, then lift your torso and legs a few inches from the floor so that your arms are straight.

- Look straight ahead and slide your shoulder blades down your back.

- Hold this position for fifteen to thirty seconds, breathing deeply throughout.

Downward Dog

- Start on the floor on your hands and knees, with your knees below your hips and your hands slightly below your shoulders. Turn your toes under in preparation to stand.

- As you exhale, lift your knees up from the floor and push your tailbone toward the ceiling.

■ On your next exhale, straighten your knees but don't lock them, and push the soles of your feet and palms of your hands into the floor.

■ Hold this position for one minute or longer, breathing deeply throughout.

Plank

■ Begin in downward dog (above). Then, as you inhale, move your torso forward so that your arms are perpendicular to the floor with your shoulders over your wrists. Your torso should be parallel to the floor, your back should be flat, and you should be looking straight down toward the floor.

■ Slide your shoulder blades down your back and lengthen your tailbone toward your heels.

■ Hold this position for thirty seconds to several minutes, breathing deeply throughout.

Child's Pose

■ Kneel on the floor with your feet together, sitting on your heels. Your knees should be hip distance apart.

■ As you exhale, lower your torso to the floor. Let your arms fall to your sides (the back of your hands will be resting on the floor and your shoulders will fall toward the floor) and rest the top of your forehead on the floor.

■ Hold this position for thirty seconds to several minutes, breathing deeply throughout.

Bridge with Block

- Lie on your back with a folded blanket or towel under your shoulders. Bend your knees so that your feet are on the floor, as close to your buttocks as possible. Your arms should be straight at your sides.

- Exhale and lift your buttocks off the floor, pressing your arms and feet into the floor. Your thighs should be parallel to your feet and the floor, and your knees should be over your heels.

- Clasp your hands together on the floor underneath your buttocks so that you stay on your shoulders.

- Hold this position for thirty seconds to one minute, breathing deeply throughout, then roll gently down to the floor.

- If you like, place a yoga block between your thighs and squeeze it as you lift your hips from the floor.

Reclining Goddess

- Lie flat on your back with your arms at your sides and lift both knees so that your feet are on the floor.

- Let your knees fall open to either side and bring the soles of your feet together. If you like, place a yoga block or rolled towel or blanket underneath each hip.

- Hold this position for a minute or two, breathing deeply throughout.

Happy Baby

- Lie on your back, exhale, and bend your knees toward your stomach.

- As you inhale, grip your feet with your hands and pull them closer to your armpits.

- As you pull in with your hands, push away with your feet, increasing the stretch.

- Hold this position for thirty seconds to one minute, breathing deeply throughout.

Bicycle

- Start on your back with your feet off the floor and your knees bent and touching your chest.

- Lace your fingers behind your head and lift your head off the floor as you inhale, keeping your chin off of your chest.

- Exhale and straighten your right leg as you bring the outside of your right arm to the outside of your left thigh.

- Inhale and return to center.

- Exhale and repeat on the other side (straighten left leg; bring outside of left arm to outside of right thigh).

- Repeat this sequence for five minutes.

Cat and Cow

- Start on your hands and knees, your back flat. Your knees should be directly below your hips and your head should be in a neutral position so that you are looking at the floor but not straining to do so.

- Exhale and round your back like a cat when it stretches, keeping your arms and knees in place.

- Inhale and return to a flat back.

- On your next inhale lift your buttocks to the ceiling and sink your stomach toward the floor (but not touching it) so your back is arched. Lift your head so that you are looking straight ahead.

- Exhale and return to a flat back again.

- Repeat this sequence ten to twenty times, breathing deeply throughout.

If you already practice yoga regularly, alone or in a class, try adding these other "sex-sational" poses to your routine: warrior, bow, boat, cow face, splits with block, rotated triangle, handstand against a wall, lunge with twists, and half moon.

DANCE PARTY!

If there's one thing my experience on *Dancing with the Stars* taught me, it's that dancing can set you free—from your doubts, fears, and hang-ups. Along with yoga, dance is one of the most important parts of my life. And even though I'm no longer competing for that big mirror ball trophy, I still try to fit some sort of dance into my day. Here's how:

- Set aside just twenty minutes for yourself, when your kids are at school, when you're on your lunch break, or when you're waiting for dinner to finish cooking. Make it clear this is your "me" time—lock the door if you must!

- Queue up the music on your stereo or MP3 player. If you're worried about the noise, use headphones. Disco and pop are great options, but play whatever music makes you feel sexy, whether that's rhumba, reggae, or Rachmaninoff.

- Get moving! Move to the music, like nobody's watching (because they're not). Or imagine that you're putting on a show for your lover—whichever scenario makes you feel least inhibited. Let go and enjoy yourself. Move your hips in circles, do some pelvic thrusts, do some pliés—say, ten hip circles to the left, ten to the right, twenty pelvic thrusts, and twenty pliés. Touch your body. Pretend you're a stripper. If you need more inspiration, play a pole-dancing DVD or even some porn to see how the "experts" move. Your goal is to free yourself of your inhibitions, worries, and tension and to put yourself in touch with your sensual side. Try it every day and see what happens!

quick study: YOGA FOR BETTER SEX?

Lisa likes to say that yoga puts her in touch with her body faster than any other type of exercise. That's not surprising: The meditative stretches and poses of yoga can help get you out of your head and in tune with your body. They're not only a great workout, but can be both calming and rejuvenating. Research even suggests that yoga may help lower blood pressure, ease symptoms of asthma, back pain, and arthritis, and prevent stroke.

But can yoga improve your sex life? A growing body of evidence suggests that the answer may be yes. Research suggests that yoga has long been used by women to benefit sexuality. And one study, published in the February 2010 issue of the *Journal of Sexual Medicine,* found that women who practiced yoga regularly for twelve weeks reported better sexual function, including improved desire, arousal, lubrication, orgasm, and satisfaction and less pain. Anecdotal reports show that some women even confess to enjoying yoga-related orgasms—or "yogasms"—during class! Yoga may help men, too: The same study found that regular yoga sessions can also benefit male sexual function, while other research has shown that it may improve premature ejaculation as well as SSRI antidepressants, a common treatment for PE.

It makes sense: Yoga requires that you regularly engage the *mula bhanda*, or the muscles in and around the genitals. These benefits can be found in any form of yoga, but kundalini yoga in particular has been shown to have tantric benefits, especially if you perform the poses with a partner. Some poses that are especially beneficial when performed with a partner are the sacred embrace, downward-facing dog, side plank, and camel. Not only do these poses improve your flexibility, but, like dance classes, they involve a lot of eye contact and nonsexual touching, making them another high-value form of foreplay. So why not take a yoga class with your sweetie? Your sex life will thank you.

good idea: BEST FOODS FOR GREAT SEX

Oysters, chocolate, red wine . . . We've all heard claims that these and other foods can pump up our sex lives. But are aphrodisiacs for real? While there's not much research into the effects of food on arousal, it's true that great nutrition can foster great sex. Certain foods and beverages—or, more accurately, the vitamins, minerals, and other compounds they contain—may indeed help improve your sex life. In general, what's good for your heart is good for your libido, because our genitals need optimal blood flow to function properly.

Why not indulge in a "sex diet" together? Cooking and eating together is a great way to bond as a couple. According to a recent survey of fifteen hundred couples, nearly 83 percent of those who said they cook together at least three times a week rate their relationship as excellent, compared to just 26 percent who said they rarely or never do. And when things heat up in the kitchen, they may start smoking in the bedroom, too: The same survey found that 58 percent of couples that often cook together are satisfied with their sex lives, compared to a third of those who don't. With that in mind, here's what's on the menu for better sex.

- **Seafood.** Oysters are the stereotypical aphrodisiac dish, possibly because they're rich in the mineral zinc, which has been linked to male fertility, potency, and sex drive. Though it may not seem quite so sexy, a humble salmon fillet may be even more important for good sex: Salmon and other fatty fish like mackerel and sardines are great sources of heart-healthy omega-3 fatty acids. Omega-3s can also help improve mood.

- **Nuts.** Some nuts, like walnuts, are high in omega-3 fats, too. Walnuts, peanuts, and cashews are also packed with L-arginine, a compound that appears to promote healthy erectile function in men and clitoral tissue in women.

- **Green veggies.** Greens in general are rich in L-arginine, while asparagus in particular is a good source of folic acid, which boosts the histamine production necessary for the ability to reach orgasm.

- **Chocolate.** We're not suggesting you scarf down a box of sweets every night, but a piece of good-quality dark chocolate may be just what the sex doctor ordered: Eating it triggers the release of the chemical phenylethylamine, leading to feelings of excitement that are conducive to sex.

part five

·

in the

BEDROOM

We believe that sex should be an integral part of a healthy lifestyle, like eating well, exercising, and brushing your teeth. First of all, great sex makes you feel good—not just while it's happening, but afterward, too. As anyone who's reveled in the afterglow knows, sex relieves stress, rejuvenates you, releases feel-good chemicals called endorphins, and improves sleep (duh). There's good evidence that regular sex has other benefits, too: Researchers at Wilkes University in Wilkes-Barre, Pennsylvania, found that people who had sex once or twice a week had higher levels of immunoglobulin A, an antibody that helps fight colds and other infections. A study published in the *Journal of Epidemiology and Community Health* found that having sex twice or more a week reduced the risk of fatal heart attack by half in men, compared with those who had sex less than once a month. Heck, sex even burns calories—about 85 calories per half-hour session. If that's not enough to inspire some nooky tonight, consider the following: Research by biological anthropologist Helen Fisher, Ph.D., suggests that people who enjoy regular sex may be more successful at work, possibly because sex can increase confidence and increase self-esteem.

Our advice: Just do it! Ian recommends that couples have sex at least once a week. We know that's not always feasible, but the key is to make an effort. Sex is a lot like exercise: It's easy to not find the time to do it, but the more you do it, the better it feels. Just like our bodies, it's easy for our sex lives to get a little flabby and we lose the desire to tone up. We tend to forget how much fun sex can be, but just having sex once a week will put you back in a regular groove, raise your testosterone levels, and resexualize your relationship. You may not be in the mood, but if you take a "try it, you'll like it attitude" and have sex at least once a week, you may find yourself suddenly making time for sex on a daily basis.

And just as a balanced diet requires variety, so does your sex life. Hey, we love chocolate as much as everyone else. But if you eat Häagen-Dazs over and over, not only will you get bored, you'll also end up depriving yourself of vital nutrients. And just like the food pyramid, there are different categories of sex that you should be "consuming" regularly: There's sex that's loving and tender and enhances emotional intimacy. There's sex for the sake of sex—because it feels good. There's sex that taps into the power of fantasy and proves that our mind is the biggest sex organ. And there's sex that plays into all of our various senses—sight, sound, touch, smell, and taste. The best sexual relationships are those that draw from all of these categories (and then some). Just think of your sex life like a salad bar: When you sample a little bit of everything, you end up feeling pretty satisfied.

That brings us to part 5 of this book, "In the Bedroom"—a tasting menu of classic sexual delights to share with your partner. Sure, you probably enjoy some dishes more than others, but there's no reason why you shouldn't mix it up every now and then. You just might surprise yourself (or your guy) by discovering new favorites.

LISA'S STORY: MY TURNING POINT

As I shared in part 1 of this book, feeling self-assured in bed wasn't always natural for me. Before I met my husband, I'd been in a couple of really toxic relationships that had turned me off to sex. Things started to change when Harry and I fell in love—and honestly, it didn't hurt that he was more experienced sexually than I was. I considered myself his willing and eager pupil!

I have to say, though, that our sex life really transformed after our girls were born. I had recently given birth to our older daughter, Delilah, and was feeling decidedly unsexy. One day I was reading the *Los Angeles Times* and came across an article about a new class called S Factor, taught by actress Sheila Kelley. The dance aspect really appealed to me, but so did the twist: The classes were a combination of ballet, yoga—and striptease. As fate would have it, Harry and I saw Sheila a few days later at a charity event. To give you an idea of how unconfident I used to feel, I had to beg Harry, who had worked with Sheila on *L.A. Law,* to ask her about the classes. I was too embarrassed.

I'm not exaggerating when I say that those classes changed my life. Sheila taught S Factor at her home, where I and other women in the small class learned how to strip, perform a lap dance, and even work the pole—all while wearing cute lingerie, sexy costumes, and "stripper heels." Yes, it was slightly terrifying at first: We were rediscovering how to move our bodies in ways that we'd been told since girlhood were "wrong," and that's a tough hang-up to lose for lots of women, including myself.

But the results were so worth it. The classes gave me a great workout, but they also strengthened the most important sex organ—my brain. I took the class for about four months (and again after the birth of my second daughter, Amelia) and came away feeling less inhibited, freer, and more confident about myself, my body, and my sexuality. I believe that being a good lover requires the right tools, and the self-esteem (and sexy moves) I gained from S Factor are permanent parts of my toolbox.

I added another tool to my bedroom arsenal a few years later—at a bachelorette party. In addition to the usual gag gifts and male strippers, there was another form of entertainment that turned out to be a real education: a woman, armed with dildos in various sizes and colors. Her name was Lou Paget, and she was there to teach us all the best tricks for satisfying a man in bed. Lou isn't how I had imagined the stereotypical "sexpert": She's classy, elegant, professional, engaging, and a whole lot of fun. After having each partygoer choose a dildo, she proceeded—with no embarrassment and in minute detail—to demonstrate all the best hand jobs and blow jobs, which she had learned from a gay friend. There were a lot of nervous giggles at first, but by the end of the evening, I had a wealth of new techniques to add to my toolbox. Lou now has a book, *How to Be a Great Lover,* which details all of these tricks. They've got cute names (Harry and I can't choose just one, but Ode to Brian, the Basketweave, Pirouette, and Seal and the Ring are some of our favorites), and Lou provides step-by-step instructions and illustrations to guide you. And keep reading—lots of saucy techniques, tips, and tricks to come!

Let's face it: The male body can be complicated, especially if you're not sure how to handle it. And while I'm all for asking your guy what pleases him, it's nice to know you have the skills to surprise—and impress—him. That's why having a sexual toolbox is so important. It's given me more confidence and fewer hang-ups, and Harry is the very happy recipient of those benefits. I feel that women are taught to feel guilty about sex ("Good girls don't do that!"), but my experiences with Sheila's and Lou's classes have taught me that we shouldn't be. Whenever someone acts shocked, I simply reply, "He's my husband." If Harry and I can't "go there" in bed, we've got a big problem.

Everyone's different, and you may not feel comfortable practicing blow jobs on a rubber penis in front of your friends or taking a stripping or pole-dancing class (which have become quite popular in recent years). But please don't give up. Any kind of dance class, whether you prefer ballroom, Zumba, or belly dance, can get you in the groove and help you start embracing your body. And the tips in this part and in part 7 can help you add lots of fun skills to your own toolbox. Now bring that newfound confidence to the bedroom!

8

UNDER THE HOOD: HIS AND HERS SEXUALITY

Ian likes to say that most men know more about what's under the hood of a car than about what's under the hood of a woman's clitoris, and he's only half joking. Of course, we can't blame guys too much: It's no secret that female sexuality is rather complex. But even though men's bodies and sex drives seem so much more straightforward, a lot of women are confused about the way they function, too. All this misunderstanding about desire and arousal can add up to some pretty unsatisfied couples—and that's before you factor in other issues such as mismatched libidos and sexual dysfunction.

That's why we've decided to give you a primer on both male and female sexuality. Even if you feel confident about your knowledge, please indulge us and take a quick read. We promise it won't be too complicated or boring, and you might even learn a few fun new facts to impress your friends.

THE BASICS OF SEXUAL RESPONSE

So let's get started with the basics. The pioneering sex researchers Masters and Johnson first developed this four-stage model for understanding sexual response in the 1960s and it still holds true today:

Excitement

Excitement starts with stimulation. That stimulation can be physical (a partner's touch, masturbation, or some other type of contact with your genitals or other part of the body), or mental and emotional (fantasy, thoughts about your partner, pornography, or simply gazing at a sexy billboard).

Whatever the cause, this stimulation causes the blood vessels in your vagina and clitoris to relax and fill with blood. In guys, the spongy tissues in the penis expand and fill with blood and he gets hard. That's not the only body part that gets erect: In both men and women, the nipples, earlobes, lips, and even nostrils also swell and darken, and your heart rate and breathing quicken and blood pressure rises.

Plateau

Excitement tends to plateau or level off before a person gets even more aroused.

As you approach orgasm, your abdomen and thighs get tense, your hands and feet clench, and your breathing becomes even quicker and more uneven. At this point, a guy will also have a full erection.

Orgasm

For many people, this third stage is the best part of sex. During orgasm, all that tension that's been building up is finally released. The physical signs that started in the plateau phase—higher blood pressure, rapid breathing, muscle contractions—kick into overdrive. But the ability to climax easily differs between men and women. All men reach a point of "ejaculatory inevitability" during sex when he can't hold back from an orgasm, no matter what. And all men have an "ejaculatory threshold," which is the amount of stimulation he can experience before reaching this "point of no return."

Women, on the other hand, don't experience ejaculatory inevitability—you can "lose" an orgasm even as it's happening. There are pros and cons to both situations: Sure, it's tougher for some women to climax, especially if they're distracted. On the other hand, women are able to enjoy multiple orgasms and have rarely been accused of coming "too fast."

Resolution

The final phase of sexual response occurs after an orgasm. For most men, this is a time to relax: The tension seeps out of his muscles, his blood pressure sinks, and his excitement dissipates. Lots of men feel sleepy during resolution and—unless he's a teenager—his penis will also take a break. This time, during which his body recovers after orgasm and he can't get another erection right away, varies depending on his age and is called the refractory period. For women, though, it's less clear cut. In fact, for some women, the first orgasm is just the start. Other women have a more malelike experience of wanting to sleep.

Sex in the Fast Lane

There's now another way of thinking about sexual arousal, thanks to a new theory developed at the Kinsey Institute by Erick Janssen and John Bancroft. Called the Dual Control Model of Sexual Response, it shows real promise for helping us understand sex. This new model for understanding sexual arousal has two parts and works the same way in men:

SEXUAL EXCITATION SYSTEM (SES). This is like the gas pedal for sexuality. Lots of things can press that pedal and rev your engine, from visual stimulation (looking at your partner, reading erotica), to tactile stimulation (having your partner touch you), and everything in between. Your SES constantly scans your environment—and your own thoughts and feelings—for things that may be sexually appealing. When it locates those things, it sends signals to your brain and genitals to activate them.

SEXUAL INHIBITION SYSTEM (SIS). Just as SES acts like the body's gas pedal, the SIS puts the brakes on your sexuality. Research suggests there are actually two different types of SIS. One responds to performance anxiety—concerns about your ability to orgasm, for example. That's called SIS-1. Your SIS-2 responds to your fear of negative consequences from sex, such as sexually transmitted diseases and unintended pregnancy. Like the SES, the SIS also constantly scans your environment, in this case for turnoffs.

ian says . . . THE JOY OF SPOONING

Sure, we all love to cuddle with our kids or pets—but what about our partners? In the beginning of a relationship, most couples love that postsex cuddle time almost as much as the act itself. Fast forward a few years, though, and we start to develop our "roll over" tendencies or even our "up and out" tendencies—whether it's to check e-mail, check on the kids, or check out that night's DVR offerings. Men have been given a bad rap for skipping out on spooning, but women are just as guilty. While it's great to have a comfy relationship where you can roll over and go to sleep—or go raid the fridge together—taking a few minutes to cuddle can make a difference. To paraphrase the pioneering sexologist Theodore Van de Velde, it's in the moments after orgasm that a man proves whether or not he's an "erotically civilized" adult. Why not be an erotically civilized couple and enjoy that afterglow in each other's arms?

We all have both an SES and an SIS—and we all need both for a healthy sex life. That makes arousal a two-part process that requires providing stimulation for the SES and removing any that might trigger the SIS. How sexually aroused you get depends on how much or how little stimulation the SES and SIS have received. Think of your sexuality as a car: You've got to have the right combination of gas and brakes for a smooth ride.

YOUR BRAIN ON SEX

According to work published by neuroscientists Ogi Ogas and Sai Gaddam in their book *A Billion Wicked Thoughts,* all it takes is a little visual stimulation to get most men in the mood for sex. That's why that lacy thong probably appeals more to your guy than to you, why he's likely got porn on his laptop, and why something like Viagra works so well for men, but not for women.

Female sexuality is a bit more complex. Sex researcher Dr. Emily Nagoski has said that "men are like driving standard transmission—if you move through the gears in the right order, you will get where you want to go—and women are like baking a soufflé: the outcome depends on the ingredients and the chef, but it also depends on the reliability of the oven, the altitude, the humidity of the day . . . more variables, more variability." Unlike guys, who tend to respond to a single trigger (say, a woman in a sexy negligee), women appear to have endless triggers for arousal. "The male sexual brain is like a single toggle switch, whereas the female sexual brain is like the cockpit of an F1 fighter jet," Gaddam has said. "There are tons of dials and instruments, and there's sophisticated calibration going on."

We really don't like to generalize when it comes to sex, and everyone is different—there are plenty of complex male "soufflés" out there, for example, while some women can get their engines revving right out of the gate. In general, though, women typically tend to have more SIS (stronger brakes) and less SES (weaker pedals) compared to men. This means that in general, women require more stimulation to become aroused, and that women are more sensitive to all kinds of threats and interruptions, from physical, to emotional, to social, than can interfere with their arousal and orgasm.

Those sensitive brakes mean that it's easy to get distracted when you want to be getting hot and heavy. Instead of focusing on your partner and your pleasure, you're busy writing mental grocery lists, planning your daughter's birthday party, or going over ideas for tomorrow's big meeting. Before you know it, you're lost in a fog of tension and stress. You can't get out of your own head, much less pay attention to his.

The solution? You need to be able to turn your brain *off* to be able to turn on sexually. In fact, scientific evidence shows that the key for women to reach the heights of orgasmic bliss is a deep sense of relaxation and a lack of anxiety. Researchers at the University of Groningen in the Netherlands scanned the brains of thirteen women and eleven men while they were manually stimulated to orgasm by their partners. The scans showed that for women, the parts of the brain responsible for processing fear, anxiety, and emotion slowed down the more aroused they became, producing a trancelike state at orgasm. Men showed far less change in these areas of the brain, suggesting that women need to relax to become aroused, while men don't. Other studies have found that women tend to fantasize more than men during sex, which also helps them escape reality and "turn off" their brains.

It's no wonder, then, that women need to do all they can to chill out and relax. Easier said than done? That's an understatement—and with busy schedules, work, kids, and everything else you've got going on, it's definitely a challenge. But by paying extra attention to the way you interact with your partner outside the bedroom, you can heat things up everywhere.

quick study: WHAT WOMEN WANT

Think you know the difference between sexual desire and arousal? You might be wrong! In fact, a number of interesting studies suggest that women can't always distinguish between their desire to have sex and their own physical arousal (increased blood flow to the genitals). According to research by University of British Columbia psychiatrist Rosemary Basson, many women are unaware of their physical arousal and don't necessarily experience sexual desire before they experience a significant amount of direct physical stimulation or have sex. For these women, Basson says, desire isn't the cause of sexual activity but the result. Guys, on the other hand, tend to be more easily aroused, and a man's arousal is more directly linked to his desire.

This concept was demonstrated—to the amusement of journalists and zookeepers alike—by Meredith Chivers of the Center for Addiction and Mental Health and J. Michael Bailey of Northwestern University. In their 2005 study, published in *Biological Psychology*, men and women watched seven two-minute clips of sex while a device measured their physical arousal (the participants also took notes about how aroused they felt). The results? All of the men, who were heterosexual, reported feeling aroused only by "straight" sex scenes—and the physiological measurements backed this up. Women, however, were far less discriminating: They also claimed to be turned on most by the heterosexual scenes, but their bodies told a different story. In fact, women were equally aroused by *all* human sexual activity—heterosexual, gay, and lesbian—and were even turned on by scenes of mating bonobo monkeys. Yep, monkeys.

Before you start worrying about whether you should trade in Tarzan for Cheetah, consider this: Previous studies by Chivers and her colleagues have shown a very low correlation between what women *say* they find arousing and their sexual arousal patterns in the lab. (This correlation is much stronger in men.) "There's the possibility that genital response for women is not necessarily imbued with meaning about their sexual interests," she explains. In other words, sometimes your vagina may act as if it has a mind of its own, but that doesn't mean you necessarily want to have sex with other women—or with monkeys, for that matter.

9

FOREPLAY, NOT "BOREPLAY"

think back to the beginning of your relationship: You probably spent some serious time just making out. To paraphrase the song, you didn't have to take your clothes off to have a good time—you and your partner were happy just to enjoy long, langorous evenings of kissing, touching, and rubbing longingly against each other as you anticipated finally having sex.

Fast-forward a few years (or ten, or twenty). These days, you're probably happy if you get any foreplay before the main event. But just like intercourse itself, foreplay can get kind of, well, routine. Sometimes it can feel as if you're both going through the motions and can predict each other's moves like clockwork. A little kissing here, a hand on a breast or penis there, some oral sex that starts to feel downright obligatory. Before you know it, the excitement and variety of foreplay has turned into "boreplay."

We can't blame you. There's something to be said for feeling comfortable—if it ain't broke, why fix it, right? But knowing exactly how to get your partner off may mean that you put less effort into turning him on, and vice versa. You forego the appetizer and go straight for the main course. And guys certainly aren't the only ones to blame. Some women just tend to assume that men don't care about foreplay, so they just skip ahead to intercourse.

The fact is that men typically orgasm more quickly, or with greater ease, than many women. The late Dr. Alfred C. Kinsey found that up to 75 percent of men ejaculate within the first few minutes of intercourse. And, as you'll learn in part 10 of this book, nearly one out of three men experience premature ejaculation.

Yet research suggests that both genders still crave a little extra attention. A 2004 study found that both women and men want more foreplay—about eighteen minutes on average. This sexual buildup is a crucial part of a healthy, satisfying sex life because it helps you become lubricated and gives him a stronger erection.

Still, many couples only enjoy a few minutes of foreplay before moving on to intercourse. Now consider that researchers from the University of Chicago have found that men reach orgasm during intercourse far more consistently than do women, and that three-fourths of men—but less than a third of women—always have orgasms as part of intercourse. The bottom line: You're not doing yourself any favors by skipping over foreplay, and you could be missing out on more opportunities for pleasure.

That's why Ian usually recommends that most couples aim for about fifteen to twenty minutes of foreplay. (We're not suggesting you incorporate a stopwatch into your bedroom routine, but you may want to pay attention to how much time has passed the first few times you try extending foreplay, just to get a general idea.) Of course, it's not just the amount of foreplay, but the quality that counts. So take the time to enjoy every moment. Bring back the mystery you once felt by keeping your clothes on for a while: A layer of fabric—whether silk, satin, cotton, or denim—between your partner's hand and your body can create all sorts of different sensations. Focus on kissing each other while slowly removing one item of clothing at a time, rather than ripping off your clothes. Want more specific suggestions for spicing up the appetizer course? Check out the ideas in this chapter.

SHOWER EACH OTHER WITH AFFECTION

A hot shower is a great way to unwind and relax after a stressful day. Now add your partner to the mix and you've got a recipe for some steamy foreplay. We also like this exercise for couples who have kids and need to steal a few moments away from the mayhem for some "we" time: Whether you simply enjoy each other's bodies while you save time (and water) with a shared shower or take things further, it's a wonderful way to reconnect.

So light some candles or dim the lights, grab some scented soap or body wash and soft washcloths, and start running that water. Then strip down with your partner and get cozy under the hot spray. Take your time soaping each other up, letting your touch linger. Your guy can give you a delicious shampoo and scalp massage while he presses his erect penis against your genitals. You can return the favor by giving your man a slow, soapy hand job. Have him place a foot on the edge of the tub, stand behind him, and rub your bare breasts against his back while you slide your hand up and down his shaft. Afterward, he can try entering you from behind, your hands against the wall or holding a securely mounted towel rack for support. But be careful: Showers can get slippery—and water can dry out your natural lubrication. It's safer to limit your shower time to foreplay, and then move things to the bedroom.

RUB-A-DUB-DUB

Like the spirit of sexy shower fun but prefer a bath? No problem. Light some candles, fill the tub, and if toys are your thing, bring a waterproof vibrator along, too. It's also not a bad idea to invest in a hose attachment for your water spout. They make for some fun underwater play, and typically cost less than ten dollars.

Let your partner get into the tub first and have him lean back against the far end of the tub, legs outstretched and slightly spread. Then carefully step into the tub and sit down between his legs with your back to him. Take a moment to enjoy the feel of your skin against his and the warmth of the water. Then your partner can slowly lather and wash you, using soft strokes on your inner thighs, your chest, your genitals, and the back of your neck before you switch places and get him nice and clean.

If you're using a toy, now's the time to play with it. Your guy can spray water at your genitals with the hose attachment, experimenting with different levels of water pressure and different angles. See if he can get you to orgasm with running water alone. Then kick things up a notch by turning on your waterproof vibrator. He can run the vibe up and down your thighs, or over your nipples, before moving south. Then it's his turn!

As the water begins to cool, drain the tub and towel each other off. You could try to have intercourse before getting out, but since water washes away your natural lubrication, the tub is really best limited to foreplay. Move on to the bedroom for the main event.

A SULTRY STRIPTEASE

Earlier, Lisa shared the story of how S Factor classes helped kick off her sexual reawakening. This exercise is inspired by her experience and is guaranteed to get a guy's engine revving—and yours, too!

First, set up a comfortable chair in the bedroom or living room, where you have room to move around as you perform. No other props are necessary—except your hot self—but if you like, get dressed up in something a little nicer than your regular clothes: Anything from demure silk jammies to a sexy cheerleader uniform with stripper heels will work, as long as you and your sweetie find it appealing.

Before you get started, remember that stripteases and lap dances aren't really about a perfect body or professional dance moves. Instead, they capitalize on teasing, anticipation, sexy moves, and the unhurried buildup of desire. So take your time: Gyrate your hips, slowly. Spin around, slowly. Bend over—*slowly*—and slap the floor before sliding your hands up your legs and gently smacking yourself on the ass. Eventually, back up into the space between his legs, facing away from him, and almost—but not quite—sit in his lap, wiggling your butt across him. Grind him slowly to an orgasm, or stop short and leave him begging for more.

BREAST ADVICE

Even if they claim to be "ass" or "leg" men, most guys we know still have plenty of love for breasts, too. Unfortunately, not every man is as skilled in the boob department as he might think: Grabbing, squeezing, pinching—there's a lot of manhandling going on above the waist! That's a shame, because the breasts are a major erogenous zone for many women.

Remember oxytocin, aka the cuddle hormone? Your body releases it when your breasts and nipples are stimulated—in fact, oxytocin is responsible for the nipple becoming erect with excitement and stimulation. As the breasts continue to receive stimulation, the body continues to release oxytocin, which has its most intense effects within the first five minutes after release, but can continue to increase contractions for up to an hour. What that means for you: more intense orgasms that feel like they involve your whole body. Also, about 1 percent of women can experience an orgasm *just* from having their breasts and nipples stimulated. Lucky ladies!

So ask your guy to take his time with your breasts. If you want to offer a little guidance and a reward at the same time, show him what you want by touching your breasts for him—you'll both come out on top.

10

TOUCHING AND TASTEFUL

find us a man who doesn't love being on the receiving end of a little oral or manual stimulation—near impossible, right? Most guys enjoy a lovingly administered hand or blow job, and you don't have to be a porn star to deliver a perfectly satisfying experience. But who wants to be average? Whether you want to brush up on your technique or honestly have no idea how to turn a man on with your hands and mouth, this chapter can help. As Lisa says, "The penis can be a pretty intimidating organ, and it's easy to feel overwhelmed by what to do with it." So allow us to share some tips to add to your sexual toolbox and take you from skittish to skilled in no time.

MALE SEXUAL ANATOMY: YOUR ROAD MAP

We all know that the stereotype is kind of true: Guys never stop to ask for directions when they're lost. Women do. So use this handy guide to navigate all the hot spots of your partner's genitals:

- **GLANS.** This is the head of the penis. It's the male equivalent of the clitoris (although the penis only has half the nerve endings of the clit).

- **CORONA.** Derived from the word meaning "crown," corona is the name of the curve at the base of the glans. This nerve-packed area is absolutely crucial to oral sex technique: Going back and forth over the "bump" of the corona, with either your mouth or your hands, provides important stimulation.

- **SULCUS.** The narrow band of skin that connects the bottom edge of the corona to the shaft is called the sulcus, and it is an extremely sensitive area.

- **FRENULUM.** This is an upside-down Y shape on the underside of the corona. If he's uncircumcised, there will be a tendonlike membrane where the foreskin connects to the shaft. If he's circumcised, this is where the foreskin used to attach to the shaft. This is the frenulum and it's incredibly sensitive.

- **SHAFT.** The shaft includes a pair of chambers, the corpora cavernosa on the top side, and the corpus spongiosum on the underside. The corpus spongiosum houses the urethra and it is very sensitive to deep pressure. All three of these chambers fill with blood as a man gets aroused. The shaft extends deep into the body. If your partner is erect, you can actually press down gently into his abdomen along the side of the penis and feel how deep it goes.

- **SCROTUM.** This is the stretchy sack of skin that envelops the testicles. Men vary in how they like to have their scrotum treated. (For ideas on how to handle it, see "Minding the Stepchildren" on page 119.)

- **TESTICLES.** Perhaps the most sensitive part of a man's reproductive anatomy, the testicles are the spongy balls inside the scrotum. Be very, very gentle with them.

- **PERINEUM.** This is the area between where the scrotum ends and the anus begins. It is sensitive to deep pressure because of its proximity to sensitive internal organs such as the prostate gland. It's also very sensitive to light touch.

- **ANUS.** The anus is a ring of muscle, densely packed with nerve endings, extremely responsive to light touch and deep pressure.

- **PROSTATE.** The prostate is very sensitive, and pressure on it results in intense, deep sensations that are totally different from penile stimulation.

ALL WET: YOUR NUMBER ONE BEDROOM ACCESSORY

Before we jump right into all the superfun stuff, we want to offer an earnest endorsement for something that's just as enjoyable—and important: lube. If you're like many women, you might assume that if you're sufficiently turned on, your body should produce all the lubrication it needs for intercourse. If you're excited, you should be wet, right? Nope.

Some women (and their partners) get discouraged if they don't produce enough natural lubrication quickly: You might start to wonder if something's wrong with you, and your guy may assume that you're just not excited by him. Neither case is usually true. It's generally easier for a woman to lubricate when she's younger or in the early stages of a new relationship. But pretty soon you get used to a certain set of stimuli, even if you're still excited. It's like your brain is telling your body, "This feels good, but I already know what's coming next." Because you might need up to fifteen minutes of stimulation before you start to lubricate and may even climax *before* you're naturally wet, we heartily recommend adding a brand of artificial lubricant to your repertoire. These products are really versatile: You can use them alone or with your partner, to increase lubrication if you experience vaginal dryness or discomfort, to help ease penetration by a penis or sex toy during vaginal or anal sex, and to spice up manual stimulation. Lubricants are also a fun way to add novelty and variety to a sexual experience, especially the flavored and warming types.

WHAT TO LOOK FOR. With so many options, shopping for lube can be a bit overwhelming. K-Y is the number one doctor-recommended brand (and Ian is both a fan and a spokesperson), but formulas vary from one brand to another; however, there are three main categories of lubricants: water based, silicone based, and oil based. Water-based lubricants are often the gentlest formulas, and are safe to use with all types of sex toys and all methods of birth control. Silicone-based lubricants are slicker and tend to last longer than water-based formulas, but may be more likely to cause irritation in some women and are not safe to use with silicone sex toys. Silicone lubricants are safe to use with most methods of birth control, with the exception of those that are also made of silicone (such as a silicone-based diaphragm or cervical cap). Oil-based lubricants are less common, as they tend to be thicker and messier than other formulas, though some people like them for their all-natural ingredients. They're unsafe to use with condoms, diaphragms, or other latex contraceptives or toys, since they can break down the materials and increase the risk of pregnancy or STD transmission. This includes products such as baby oil, olive oil, and body cream.

HOW TO USE. There's no reason that applying lubricant has to be awkward. In fact, you can make it a sexy part of foreplay. Start with a small amount of lubricant, about the size of a dime or nickel. Depending on the type of sexual activity you're engaging in, apply lubricant directly to the vulva, just inside the vagina, or to the anus. If you're using condoms, you can apply lubricant to the outside of the condom, which will help with penetration and add sensation for your guy. (Never apply lubricant on the shaft of the penis before wearing a condom, since the condom could slip off. Lubricant should be limited to the reservoir tip of the condom.) If you're using a sex toy, you can apply lube directly to the toy or to the area of the body it's being used in or on. Remember, if you're using a water-based lubricant, you may need to reapply it a few times, since the body easily absorbs these formulas. Silicone-based formulas tend to last longer. Most important, make using a lubricant fun and give yourself a chance to get used to it.

KEEP IN MIND. Remember, anything that comes into contact with a woman's genitals can cause infection or irritation, by interrupting the natural bacteria balance that fights off infection or simply as a result of ingredients that your body is sensitive to. Some women are more sensitive than others. As a rule, you should always test a new lubricant on a small patch of skin and leave it for twenty-four hours before applying it to the genitals. Flavored lubricants may be especially likely to promote irritation or infection, as they often contain sugar.

A SLIPPERY ISSUE

Trying to conceive? You may need to pass up using a lubricant. A 2005 study presented at the American Society for Reproductive Medicine found that several popular lubricants decrease the chances of conception. Use of a lubricant slowed down sperm and also decreased the quality of the sperm, interfering with their ability to reach and fertilize an egg. In particular, the study found that Replens slowed sperm down by 89 percent, while Astroglide did so by 60 percent. Two other formulas, FemGlide and K-Y Jelly were less harmful, slowing sperm down by 15 percent and 10 percent, respectively. However, not all lubricants have been tested in relation to whether they slow down the movement of sperm. Couples who prefer to use a lubricant may want to try PreSeed, a lubricant designed just for those trying to conceive. Researchers found no significant differences in how fast sperm moved with PreSeed.

GIVE HIM A HAND

Hand jobs? Aren't those a little . . . *retro?* Something you do when you're a teenager and leave behind along with your virginity? We couldn't disagree more. Manual and oral stimulation are at the heart of pleasuring, and—as Lisa described earlier—the humble hand job is just one more tool for you in your toolbox of sexual options. After all, any one method of stimulation is bound to get boring after a while. A great hand job is just that: yet another way to bring pleasure to your partner.

Worried that you won't do as good a, er, job as he could do himself? Ask him to show you what he likes. As we'll discuss in part 8, the increased accessibility of Internet porn means that men are masturbating more often. As a result, a guy can develop what's called an idiosyncratic masturbatory style: He's become so accustomed to the specific way *he* touches his penis that it can be difficult to climax through regular intercourse. By demonstrating exactly how he masturbates, he can give you a good idea of how to give him a successful hand job. He'll probably appreciate that you want to learn how to please him. As Ian says, "Most guys think there's something awfully nice about getting a hand job from someone other than themselves." A little enthusiasm goes a long way, so read up on technique, grab a bottle of lube, and start experimenting!

SHOW AND TELL. A little show and tell will help educate you about your man's pleasure and leave you both satisfied. Lie in bed next to each other, start touching yourself, and encourage your guy to do the same. It may feel weird doing something that's typically a private pleasure in front of someone else, but if you allow yourself to relax, you may find yourself enjoying it. If you feel comfortable enough, try gazing into his eyes as you pleasure yourself, which will increase your connection.

After the two of you have been doing this for a while, take turns touching each other. Rest your hand lightly on top of his, guiding him to the best ways to get you off, and vice versa. Run your fingers over his testicles, and up and down the sides of his shaft. Place your palm over the head of his penis and move your hand in a twisting motion, as if you're squeezing juice from a lemon. Then move on to some firm upward stroking. Or stroke downward on his shaft, alternating hands so that the friction is constant. You can take him to orgasm and make this the main event, or step back and move on to intercourse.

RUB HIM THE RIGHT WAY. A hand job can be a quick, isolated surprise (think dark, empty movie theater or parked car), but it can also be just one aspect of a long, languorous evening that focuses on the pleasure of touch. For the latter, you just need a bottle of massage oil and some time. To start, have your guy lie down on his stomach, with his arms at his sides. Kneel beside him, and run your hands firmly down the length of his body, all the way from the upper back down to the tips of his toes. Do this several times, adding in the massage oil. Begin massaging your partner's back. Kneeling above his head, place your palms on his upper back, facing downward, and push them all the way down to the buttocks, then out to either side and up to the shoulders. Massage the shoulders, pulling your hands up from the front to the back. Next, place your hands on the upper back with your hands palm to palm, like you're praying, and repeat the motions you made when your hands were palms down. Make small circles with your thumbs up and down the sides of the spine, and then massage the sides of the torso by pulling upward with your palms. Slide your hands up and down his legs; then do the same with his arms. Ask him to roll over, and repeat the arm and leg massages from the front. Don't forget his feet.

Now it's time to focus on his genitals. Start by stroking his shaft in an upward motion. Then, place one hand at the base of the penis, while placing your other hand palm down on the head, as if you were squeezing a lemon. Stroke the shaft up and down with the one hand while using the other hand to massage the head in a circular motion. Keep rubbing him to climax (and then ask him to return the favor!) or transition into intercourse if you prefer.

LET YOUR FINGERS
DO THE TALKING

As Lisa learned, the ability to give your guy a stellar hand job can boost your confidence in bed—and keep him coming back for more. These variations are adapted from recommendations by Good in Bed contributor and sex educator Dr. Emily Nagoski, author of *The Good in Bed Guide to Orally Pleasuring a Man*. Try them on your man and watch him swoon with pleasure.

THE JUICER. With his penis pointing straight out, place your fingertips around the corona as though you're going to pluck it. Move your hand up and twist your wrist, like you're juicing a lemon or an orange. You can also try it without the twist. All you need is a very light touch.

INFINITE VAGINA. He'll need a pretty firm erection for this one. With your hands well lubed, wrap your hand around the head of his penis and stroke down. Follow that hand immediately with your opposite hand. Keep alternating, following one hand with the other, so the head of his penis is constantly being stimulated with a downward motion. Guys describe this as feeling like penetration that goes on forever. A related technique (reverse vagina) involves pulling up with your hands instead of stroking down.

CLOCK. With your hands working the reverse vagina, gently tug his penis so it's pointing toward his navel. Then rotate the penis gradually clockwise, so that with each stroke the head points around over to the hipbone, then down to his knees, then around to the other hipbone, and back up to the navel.

PEACE. Make a V with your index and middle fingers, like you're making a peace sign, and stroke the glans and shaft between those fingers. (With guys with particularly thick penises, this might be a bit more difficult.) This will produce light touch sensations—those fingers just aren't strong enough to produce deep touch in that position—so it's especially nice around the glans and corona. With your fingers in that position, you can try brushing the webbing at the base of your fingers against his frenulum.

UPSIDE DOWN. Lying next to your guy, rather than holding his penis in the traditional fashion, flip your hand upside down so your thumb is on the underside. This might feel awkward to you, but your partner may find he really enjoys it.

BLOW HIS MIND

If there's one sex act that women seem to disagree about, it's fellatio: Some of you love performing it, while others find it an unappealing chore. In fact, surveys suggest that men enjoy receiving oral sex more than women enjoy performing it. Yet, done well, fellatio can be a pleasurable option, whether it's a regular part of your routine, you're surprising your guy with it, or you rely on it as an alternative during times when you're just not up for intercourse. At its best, a good blow job requires a healthy dose of trust and imagination on the part of both you and your partner. By following the tips in this section, you may learn to love giving oral sex or simply kick your skills up several notches if you're already a fan.

Overcoming Your Reservations

There's a reason why they call it a "job": Even the most enthusiastic fellators know that the best blow jobs take some effort. If you're absolutely against oral sex, though, we heartily encourage you to reconsider: With a few simple tricks, you can make the process not just tolerable but enjoyable:

■ Some people are hesitant to put someone's genitals in their mouth. Mostly genitals are like any other body part, and if you feel comfortable kissing his lips or his shoulders or his belly, you can feel comfortable kissing his genitals. Worried about hygiene? Take a shower together first.

■ For some women, fears of gagging or bad past experiences have turned them off to fellatio. Gagging happens when something, in this case the penis, hits the back of the throat. It also can happen for psychological reasons, however—just the thought of an erect penis going into the mouth can trigger fear or disgust, which may lead to gagging. One solution for gagging during fellatio, no matter when it occurs, is to regain a sense of control over what's happening. Porn films like *Deep Throat* have led many women to mistakenly believe that good technique requires taking as much of the penis as possible into the mouth—and this is definitely *not* true. Instead, you can ease your way into fellatio with licking or taking only the glans (head) of the penis into the mouth, which also happens to be the most sensitive spot. Putting one or both of your hands on his shaft can help create the sensory illusion that more of the penis is in your mouth, and allows you to control the depth and rhythm and movement. Often, the gag reflex fades away as you begin to enjoy it as much as the person receiving it. There are no rules, so have fun and do only what feels good and comfortable.

■ Don't do it just because he wants it. That's a martyr blow job, and it doesn't make either of you very satisfied.

■ Experiment cautiously. Try a few of the tips and techniques here. Remember, there's no obligation, and the fact that you're looking for ways to learn to love fellatio is great in itself.

■ To swallow or not to swallow? There's no rule that says you must swallow his ejaculate when performing fellatio or that this decision means anything about your feelings for him. Whether because you don't like the taste of semen or fear sexually transmitted infections, it is entirely a personal preference. If you don't like to swallow, you can finish your guy with manual stimulation, let the ejaculate land elsewhere, or switch to intercourse—and that's just fine. At that point, he should be so wrapped up in his orgasm that whether or not you swallow should be the least of his concerns.

What *shouldn't* you do? Well . . .

- Watch your teeth—no biting (unless he's told you that's his thing). Keep your nails filed smooth and take off any rings before you start.

- Don't let up on the pressure. You'd be surprised by how much pressure a penis can take. Try a wide range of intensities, including things you're not really sure he'll respond to. Experiment.

- Enjoy yourself. If fancy tricks aren't your style, leave the deep throating to porn stars. They're getting paid.

- Be in the moment. Even quiet guys give out tons of signals about what they like. If he's holding his breath, gasping, or huffing, he's feeling pretty darn good. As his arousal increases, his abdomen, thighs, and buttocks will contract, and as he approaches orgasm his scrotum will tighten. The worst things you can do during a blow job are to look grossed out or bored. If you'd rather be watching *Grey's Anatomy,* you should just go do that and save fellatio for another time.

Oral Options

These tricks are also inspired by Ian's colleague Emily Nagoski, Ph.D. (Although Ian has only received oral sex from one woman for about as long as he can remember, he—and his wife—consider Emily to be their guru on the subject!) Her advice can take you from blow-job beginner to a seasoned pro in no time.

SLOW DANCE. This technique is a great way to bring your man to attention, fast. While his penis is still soft, get as much of it in your mouth as you can and then slowly and gently, but firmly, suck and draw your head upwards so that his penis stretches. Draw your lips up to the head. You can allow his penis to slip out of your mouth and then start over, or you can keep it in your mouth and go back down to go again. Rest your hand on his inner thigh, lower abdomen, or scrotum for an additional sensation.

VACUUM. Open your mouth wide enough to accommodate his penis and plunge your mouth down as far as you feel comfortable; then come back up. Concentrate exclusively on the head, with your lips never leaving the glans, or keep your lips low on the shaft and brush the glans against your soft palate or the roof of your mouth.

FRAPPE. With your hand wrapped around the base, wrap your lips around the head of the penis. Suck like you're trying to slurp a really thick milk shake through a straw. This is great when he's erect, but you might also find that if you do it when he's still soft, it will make him hard pretty fast.

TONGUE STRUM. Extend your tongue out of your mouth and flick it up and down as fast as you can. You can do this up and down the length of the shaft, or you can focus on the frenulum.

SWIRL. As you go down, swirl your tongue in a half circle around the frenulum, and as you go up, complete the circle. Use it in combination with a wrist twist to drive him wild.

CREAMSICLE. Imagine that his penis is your favorite frozen dessert on a stick and then lavish it with the same attention. Bonus: This treat is calorie free!

POWERHOUSE. With your hand wrapped around his shaft so that your index finger is around the sulcus, put your mouth over the head. Your lips will touch your index finger. Using lots of saliva, suck just the glans, moving mouth and hand in unison so that your fingers brush over the frenulum as your lips reach the tip of the glans, going up and down in tight, wet motions.

HOT AND COLD. Take a mug of hot (not boiling) water and a glass of ice water. With a little mouthful of ice water, slip your mouth over his erect penis and swirl your tongue around the head and shaft. Then take a sip of hot water and repeat. Keep alternating. It probably won't push him over the edge, but it will definitely keep his attention.

MINDING THE STEPCHILDREN

Lisa always gets a chuckle from this euphemism, which refers to a man's scrotum and testicles: As Lou Paget has said, "They're like stepchildren—they tend to be ignored!" If you don't know how your guy feels about having his scrotum touched (and if you haven't asked, you don't know—just because he hasn't actively asked for it doesn't mean he's not interested), there are loads of techniques you can try. Here are some favorites:

1. Lightly stroking the scrotum provides gentle, teasing stimulation and is a great accompaniment to oral sex.

2. Licking the scrotum also provides a light sensation that many guys really enjoy.

3. Light touch and warmth are the main sensations that stimulate the scrotum. But you've got to handle his scrotum carefully.

ian says . . . DO MEN LIKE GIVING ORAL SEX?

As a sex counselor, I'm often asked whether men really enjoy giving a woman oral sex or if it's more of a chore they grudgingly offer either in hopes of receiving fellatio or to return the favor afterward. This couldn't be further from the truth. As the author of *She Comes First* (an entire book that's basically one long ode to the joys of cunnilingus), I can honestly say that the vast majority of men that I've spoken with take a gung-ho attitude when it comes to going down on their female partners.

In fact, many men complain that they're not the ones with the issue. As it turns out, many women worry that guys don't really enjoy going down, or you worry that you're taking too long, or that your smell/taste might be unappealing. Many women also have a low sense of genital self-esteem, and feel like their vulvas are not necessarily their most attractive feature. Rather than worry that a guy might not be into going down, instead focus on how to give him constructive feedback. Let him know what feels good and what doesn't. It's always okay to tell a guy to be gentler, or to slow down, or to keep doing what he's doing—we tend to get a little overexcited.

If you have a guy who's a little shy, you can always tell him that you had a sexy dream about him, and when he asks you what you dreamed about, be sure to include some long-lasting cunnilingus in your description. But if your guy needs a little nudge, then give him one. Literally. Gently push his head in a southerly direction during foreplay. And if he is one of those men who likes to get more than give, or has some old-school ideas about feminine hygiene, then it's time to set him straight. He needs to know that the vagina is a self-cleaning ecosystem, and that when it comes to female orgasm, the tongue is mightier than the sword.

try this: TALK DIRTY TO ME

Remember that episode of *Seinfeld* in which Jerry's date responded with horror to his bedroom banter? "You were the one who was talking dirty!" he shouts after her as she storms off. "I was just trying to keep up!"

As Jerry learned, talking dirty in bed can be tricky: Go too far and you run the risk of scaring off your partner—or, more likely, feeling silly. Yet a few well-placed utterances can go a long way to spicing things up between the sheets. That makes sense, since speaking or hearing erotically charged words triggers the production of the feel-good novelty-generated neurotransmitter dopamine. Do it right with these tips:

KEEP IT SIMPLE. No need to mimic porn star dialogue, unless that turns you both on. Short, not-so-sweet nothings can give an even more powerful punch. Your basic, "Ooh, yeah" may work just fine.

COMPLIMENT YOUR PARTNER. Statements like "You're so hot" and "You taste so good" can get you going and boost your partner's confidence.

SAY WHAT YOU LIKE. If your partner is turning you on, tell him: You'll not only reinforce great behavior, but saying the words can help you focus on the action as it's happening—particularly important for women, who can tend to get distracted during sex. "That feels great," "I love it when you lick my nipples," "Keep touching me there . . ." If you like it, say so.

FINISH STRONG. While we're not fans of ongoing commentary on the action—you're not a sportscaster, after all—two simple words can send your partner over the edge. About to orgasm? Tell your man, "I'm coming!" Guys tend to view a woman's orgasm as a badge of honor. Not only are you telling him he's doing something really, really right, but you're also giving him permission to climax himself.

good idea: TOP-TEN TIPS FOR
MIND-BLOWING FELLATIO

The difference between good oral sex and great oral sex is as simple as these top-ten tips, courtesy of Dr. Emily Nagoski:

- **Get him wet.** Just like hand jobs and intercourse, a stellar blow job requires lubrication. Use saliva or experiment with flavored lubes.

- **Use your hands.** They have more strength and stamina than your mouth ever will, so much of the stimulation of a blow job will come from your hands. Use your fingers, palm, and wrist to do the work that your tongue, lips, and jaw can't.

- **Use your tongue, too.** Lick. Flick. Brush. Even if these things don't make him climax, they're different from what he'll experience during any other kind of sex, and novelty is a good thing.

- **Put the squeeze on.** Squeeze a little as you move your hand up, release as you move your hand down. And twist your wrist.

- **Suck it.** Suction is a special feature of oral sex that neither intercourse nor a hand job can replicate. With practice your jaw will strengthen so you can suck harder and longer, but in the meantime, suck gently, saving the really intense sucking for the pivotal moment.

- **Keep a steady rhythm.** When you find the pace that makes him sigh and shiver, stick with it.

- **Don't just focus on his penis.** The best blow jobs combine stimulation of the penis with the scrotum, perineum, anus, rectum, prostate, thighs, belly, nipples, and whatever else you can reach. The idea is to swirl him upward in a whirlwind of sensations until his eyes cross and his toes curl.

- **Be confident.** A "Wow, she really knows what she's doing!" response doesn't come from technique but from attitude.

- **Pay attention.** The more attention you pay, the more attuned you'll be to the clues his body is sending you about his arousal state. With practice, you'll learn to read his signals intuitively.

- **Love what you're doing—or act like it.** Masturbate while you go down. Make noise. Make eye contact. Enjoy the feel of his penis in your hands and mouth and you cannot go wrong.

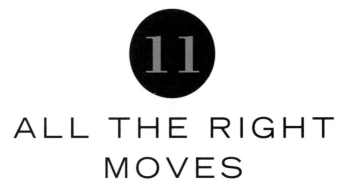

ALL THE RIGHT MOVES

Intercourse is the main sexual event for most couples, and for good reason: Few things can make you feel as close to your partner. While intercourse is usually pleasurable for both parties, it's not always the best path to orgasm for women. In fact, the physiological aspects of intercourse definitely favor male orgasm. Just one-third of women regularly reach orgasm during intercourse. Another third need added direct stimulation of their clitoris to climax, and the final one-third find it's easier to orgasm from other types of sexual activity—whether manual or oral stimulation, sex toys, or other types of sex play—or have trouble reaching orgasm altogether.

It's a sad consequence of anatomy that many intercourse positions don't directly stimulate a woman's clitoris. Fortunately, there's a lot you can do to up your odds of orgasmic bliss. If you're able to reach orgasm through other types of stimulation (such as masturbation, manual stimulation, or oral sex), but not during intercourse, try adding some direct clitoral stimulation to intercourse. You or your partner can use one or two fingers to rub your clitoris during intercourse. A small vibrator works well, too, especially bullet vibrators that can be attached to a penis ring for hands-free stimulation. We'll talk more about these toys in part 7.

We also recommend trying out different positions during sex. Some of these are particularly good for increasing your chance of orgasm. So start experimenting! Who knows? You might just find some new favorites.

MISSIONARY

If sexual positions were ice cream flavors, the missionary (also known as male superior, or man on top) would certainly be vanilla. But a lot of us love vanilla—especially if it's made with gourmet Tahitian vanilla beans and not artificial flavoring! In other words, missionary doesn't have to mean boring.

HOW TO: Simple—your guy gets on top of you. Spice it up by adding a pillow under your hips to help him stimulate your G-spot. If you enjoy deep penetration (and are somewhat flexible), you can rest your ankles on his shoulders.

PROS: Excellent for maintaining eye contact with your partner. The missionary position is one of the most common sexual positions—and there's something to be said for comfort and routine.

KEEP IN MIND: It's difficult for many women to orgasm in missionary. Add some clitoral stimulation with your finger or a toy, or use this position after you've already climaxed.

WOMAN ON TOP

Also known as female superior, this is a favorite among many couples, and no wonder: It's the position that most consistently leads to female orgasm.

HOW TO: He lies on his back and you straddle him.

PROS: Gives your guy an excellent view of your breasts and clitoris and allows you both to stimulate them easily. Increases your chances of orgasm, since you control the angle and depth of penetration, and may also stimulate the G-spot in some women. Woman on top is also a good option if your partner has premature ejaculation because it ups your odds of climaxing even if he can't last long (more on this in part 10).

KEEP IN MIND: This position takes the work off your guy's shoulders and puts it on yours (or your thighs, to be exact). Most men love it for that very reason, but it can be quite a workout for you, depending on how rigorous you get. Think of it as a fun way to burn some calories.

CAT

Short for coital alignment technique, this variation on the missionary position is designed to provide direct, hands-free stimulation of the clitoris during vaginal intercourse by pressing you and your partner pelvis to pelvis. Meow!

HOW TO: You wrap your legs around your man and he uses slow, deeper thrusts while making sure that his pelvic bone rubs against your vulva and clitoris. The focus here is grinding and rocking back and forth.

PROS: Places your clitoris in the middle of the action, so it increases your ability to climax from intercourse.

KEEP IN MIND: Your clit and vulva need to be in constant contact with his pelvic bone for this position to be its most mind-blowing.

REVERSE COWGIRL

This position allows for G-spot stimulation, as well as easy stimulation of your breasts, thighs, abdomen, vulva, and clitoris. Ride him, cowgirl.

HOW TO: You sit on him as in woman on top, but face his feet.

PROS: Reverse cowgirl hits a lot of your hot spots, plus it allows you or your partner to stimulate even more areas.

KEEP IN MIND: Like woman on top, reverse cowgirl is more physically strenuous for you. We think the results are worth it.

SPOONING

The side-by-side nature of this position makes it great for intimacy—plus, it's easier on your back and your partner's.

HOW TO: You and your partner lie on your sides so that he's "spooning" you from behind.

PROS: Spooning is comfortable but it's also a turn-on: You can synchronize your movements and you have more ability to control your guy's penis, using it to stimulate you where you want. He can also reach around to touch your clitoris and breasts.

KEEP IN MIND: Because spooning is so slow and easy, it's great for longer sex sessions, but it's also a good choice for couples coping with premature ejaculation, since it's easy for the man to pull out and press the head of his penis to delay his orgasm. (See chapter 18 for details.)

REAR ENTRY

Yup, doggy style. Not every woman is a fan of this position—some view it as too "animalistic" or miss the ability to gaze into their partner's eyes. If that sounds like you, we respectfully ask you to reconsider: Rear entry can provide both of you with just enough friction and pressure to prove that there's nothing wrong with doing it like they do it on the Discovery Channel.

HOW TO: There are several variations on this position: In one of the most popular, you're on your hands and knees while your partner stands or kneels behind you. You can also lie facedown or with a pillow under your hips, which takes the strain off your guy's knees and legs while stimulating your G-spot.

quick study: IS THE G-SPOT FOR REAL?

The existence of the so-called G-spot has long been a source of controversy among experts—right up there with elusive creatures like the Loch Ness monster and Bigfoot (but, let's face it, a lot sexier). A number of scientists believe that stimulating this sensitive area of the vagina—typically located one to three inches up the front vaginal wall between the vaginal opening and the urethra—can produce increased sexual arousal and stronger orgasms for some women. Yet not everyone agrees.

The G-spot has been studied since the 1940s, although its name—a nod to German gynecologist Ernst Gräfenberg—wasn't coined until 1981. Since then, we've been bombarded with seemingly countless magazine articles and research studies, either offering advice for stimulating this pleasure spot or debating its existence in some, or all, women. And the disagreement doesn't appear to be ending anytime soon: A small 2010 study published in the *Journal of Sexual Medicine* found that some women who reported having powerful orgasms had a thicker area of vaginal tissue than their peers. Yet another larger 2010 study in the same journal found no definitive evidence of the G-spot's existence. Other researchers suggest that the G-spot may actually be an interior extension of the clitoris.

PROS: Classic rear entry (you on all fours) gives your guy a great view, allows you or him to stimulate your breasts and clitoris, and we can't deny that there's something deliciously dirty about doggy style. When you lie down or support your hips on a pillow, you give his penis even better access to your G-spot, which can trigger a whole different set of sexy sensations.

KEEP IN MIND: It's not the most romantic position, but rear entry lets your man thrust more deeply, a bonus for guys dealing with delayed ejaculation (see part 10 for details). For that reason, rear entry is a good choice to wrap up a night of lovemaking.

Whatever the studies say, some positions do seem to stimulate this hot spot in some women, so it's worth giving them a trial run to see if that holds true for you. In general, you want to try positions that shallowly stimulate the top wall of the vagina (the side closest to your belly button). Engaging in some manual stimulation with fingers or toys prior to intercourse is also a good way to explore.

- Woman-on-top position allows you to lean forward or backward, depending on the shape of your partner's penis, to stimulate this area.

- Reverse cowgirl position can also help, particularly if his penis points slightly downward. This also gives you control so you can move around to find the most pleasurable angle.

- Propping a pillow under your lower back during missionary position is usually the best way to reach the G-spot, as it angles your vagina on a downward slant, making this area more accessible with penetration.

- Facedown rear entry is another effective position, in which you lie flat on the bed while he enters you from behind, again experimenting with depth and angle of penetration.

ian says . . . THE JOY OF COMFORT SEX

Sex with your significant other is a bit like ordering dinner from your favorite take-out restaurant: Sure, it's predictable, but the meal always tastes good and satisfies your hunger.

Just as there's comfort food, there's also comfort sex, whose virtues are completely underrated. Our culture is obsessed with all things new and fresh, and sex is no exception, from magazine headlines promoting the latest, greatest positions, to our tendency to trade in old partners for newer, more exciting models.

But in my opinion, the tried and true often has distinct advantages—especially when it comes to sex. First, many women don't even experience orgasm the first few times they have sex with a man, which may have an evolutionary basis: Because the female orgasm usually comes more slowly than the male orgasm, its mastery requires dedication and patience, which encourages you to seek out a man who will ultimately invest adequate time and energy to familiarize himself with your unique sexuality.

This "getting to know you" process of familiarization extends into long-term relationships as well. And that's where comfort sex can really benefit you. When it comes to ensuring orgasm, predictability is a good thing. Sexual arousal involves both voluntary and involuntary physiological processes: Orgasm itself is an involuntary response to voluntary sexual stimulation.

BEND ME, SHAPE ME: EXPANDING YOUR HORIZONS

The basic positions we've described here are all many couples need or want for satisfying sex. And if you're like a lot of people, you're perfectly happy sticking to a tried-and-true bedroom routine, as long as it ends with both of you happy. Maybe you've got a few key go-to positions and occasionally mix it up with one of the other classics. After all, there's something to be said for the virtues of "comfort sex," as Ian describes above.

Comfort sex promotes the seamless transition from the voluntary to the involuntary: You know where you're going, so you don't have to think about it—you can just let go and enjoy your pathway to orgasm. Neurologically, when your brain becomes familiar with a process, you're no longer relying on the prefrontal cortex to learn new things, but instead are letting those routines get imprinted into your basal ganglia, a part of the brain that does not require conscious thought.

Anytime you introduce newness or novelty into your sex life, you are making the prefrontal cortex learn and adapt, which means you're thinking about what you're doing while you're doing it. This makes it harder to cross that voluntary/involuntary threshold and just let go. For some people, the result is "spectatoring," or worrying about sex while they're having it. With comfort sex, you know what works and have a sex script or two that you and your partner like to follow. Predictable? Yes, but also pleasurable—especially if you tend to have a hard time achieving orgasm.

Of course, it's only natural for couples to get bored, lose interest in sex, or look for ways to spice things up. Novelty and newness absolutely have their place, but don't confuse the predictable routines of comfort sex with boredom. Instead, keep your sex script fresh by introducing novelty in foreplay: Share a fantasy, try some role-playing, take a sexy shower together, or explore something kinky together—check out part 7 of this book for plenty of suggestions. Whatever you decide, use novelty to enhance desire and jump-start the process of arousal, and then let yourselves fall back on the familiarity that you know will get you to orgasm.

But what if you're one of those couples who crave constant variety? What if the classics make you stifle a yawn? What if you're a pair of thrill seekers, eager to experiment with something a little more . . . acrobatic?

Well, we can help with that, too. These days, there's no shortage of books, DVDs, websites, and even smartphone apps devoted to the latest and greatest sexual positions. To start, though, we'd like to recommend the *Kama Sutra*. This ancient Hindu love manual was once considered valuable for its psychological insights on love and relationships, though most people today know it as a how-to

HOME, SWEET HOME

Whether you live in a studio apartment or a mansion, you still have some sexually undiscovered territory in your home. Mix up the scenery by christening these spots.

BEDROOM. Ease your way out of bed and get frisky on a bedroom chair or in front of a full-length or vanity mirror.

BATHROOM. Your tub and shower can set the stage for fabulous foreplay, but we recommend saving intercourse for afterward, as water tends to wash away a woman's natural lubrication. Plus, there's nothing sexy about showing up at the ER after a sex-induced slip-and-fall. Men can also bend their partners over the sink for a private quickie.

DINING ROOM. Sweep those dishes onto the floor (or, for a less-destructive option, make sure the table is bare) and get passionate. Armless chairs are also great choices for woman-on-top positions or for sexy lap dances.

DOOR JAMB. A door frame can give you some much-needed support during rush-home-and-rip-your-clothes-off standing sex.

KITCHEN. Try out the countertop—just stay clear of the stove.

LIVING ROOM. The couch is a natural nooky spot for movie-night canoodling, but also consider chairs, ottomans, the floor, the coffee table . . . just do a good cleanup before you have guests.

PORCH. Your sunporch, lanai, balcony, or deck can give you that feeling of public sex with less risk. Be wary of neighbors and traffic if you live in a busy area.

sex text. In reality, only one section of the book focuses on sexual intercourse—but it's still quite useful if you're in search of alternative sexual positions.

There are a number of modern *Kama Sutra* books out there worth trying. Among them: *Kama Sutra 52* contains a year's worth of positions—one for each week. *Kama Sutra Step by Step* offers photographic instructions of different positions, including a number of variations and enhancements. And Nerve's *Position of the Day Playbook* has a position for every single day of the year. We suggest choosing a book and flipping through it together, bookmarking the positions you find most intriguing.

It's all about personal preference, but to start you might want to try a variation of the missionary position, in which he enters you and then rocks his body in order to assist you in bringing your legs pressed together within his. This position makes it possible for your vulva and clitoris to be stimulated during penetration, hugging your guy's genitals between your legs. Another hot option requires the man to sit in a chair with his legs relaxed. You face him and straddle him with your feet on the floor. You then slowly lower yourself onto his erect penis. This one is great, because it offers a maximum of upper body—and eye—contact and also allows you total control over both the speed and depth of your partner's thrusting. These are two of the easiest *Kama Sutra* positions. Some positions may require more practice, but the effort will be well worth it.

You might also want to experiment with tantric sex. Popularized by devotees such as the pop star Sting, tantric sex is really just an aspect of a religious philosophy in which practitioners seek to harness the divine power that flows through the universe (including their bodies) in order to attain their goals. Sexually, couples can use tantra to become more attuned to each other, and experience longer, more intense, and more satisfying sexual sessions.

Set the mood by lowering the lights, lighting candles, and even playing some soft music. Relax by showering together, or give each other massages, or even share a glass of wine and chat. Then, sit across from each other and gaze into each other's eyes, and try to match your breathing to your partner's for about five or ten minutes.

Next, caress each other's bodies and discuss what feels good. As you transition into foreplay, continue to harmonize your breathing and maintain eye contact. Move into slow, sensual sex, using mindfulness and the exercising of your pelvic muscles to hold off on your orgasm. If you feel yourself getting ready to climax, pause, relax, tighten your pelvic muscles, and breathe. Then continue for as long as you can manage. While quick and dirty sex is hot, the slow sensuality of tantric sex can take your pleasure to new heights.

try this: THE ART OF THE QUICKIE

Feel as if you and your partner don't have time for a lengthy lovemaking session? Try a quickie or two. Revered by parents, workaholics, and otherwise busy couples, the quickie is an excellent way to reconnect while boosting your libido and warding off the dreaded sex rut. Here's how to make it count:

Start slow: Approach your guy from behind as he's washing dishes or working at the computer. Slide your hands over his shoulders and give him a quick massage before turning him around and delivering a deep and lingering kiss. When you sense he might want more, end the kiss and walk away.

Later on, once the kids are tucked away in bed, indulge in some heavy petting with your guy. Explore each other's bodies with your hands, taking care to avoid the hot spots for now. Touch just enough to leave both of you feeling on edge. Let your partner know that you'd be up for more a little later on. Surprise him when he's on the phone or otherwise preoccupied by pulling him close and sliding a hand down his pants. Place a firm hand around his penis, letting your fingers glide up and down the shaft as much as possible. Reach down farther to cup his testicles and place your palm over the head of his penis and rub.

At this point, you'll probably both be awfully hot and bothered. So just unzip him and pull aside your panties. You can lift your leg, allowing your partner to support you by the thigh to allow for greater ease of penetration. The frenzy of a quickie can be an incredible turn-on, and the levels of arousal you build up throughout the day should make that final release plenty satisfying for both of you.

SEXY STAYCATIONS

There's no doubt that vacation sex is smokin'. But you don't need to leave home to harness that chilled-out, carefree feeling. In fact, some experts believe that the positive emotions associated with out-of-town lovemaking may linger even longer than typical post-vacation relaxation. Reap the benefits with sensual "staycations" aimed at reconnecting with your partner. Here are three of our favorites.

Tropical Staycation

Love the laid-back vibe of "island time" but can't afford a week in Fiji or a getaway to St. Martin? No worries! It's easy to re-create that tropical aura at home.

SET THE SCENE: If the weather is warm, kick things off with a trip to your local beach, pool, or water park or lounge in your yard under an umbrella. Don't despair if it's the dead of winter, though. Turn up the heat, don a bathing suit, and spread a few towels on the living room rug. Play a mix of Caribbean tunes or, if you prefer something more relaxing, the sounds of gentle waves. Mix up some margaritas or piña coladas in the blender. Light a few scented candles for the aroma of fresh ocean water, coconuts, or tropical flowers. Depending on your budget, you might even add a few inflatable palm trees, festive lanterns, and orchids.

THE PLAN: Isn't there something so delicious about the feel of your lover's warm hands rubbing suntan lotion into your skin? Use that experience as inspiration for your own sensual rubdown, substituting high-quality massage oil for the sunscreen. Invite your partner to relax facedown on a beach towel while you open the bottle of oil. Next, kneel beside him, pour some oil into your palms, and run your hands firmly down the length of his body, from the upper back to the tips of his toes. Make sure you cover all those beautiful body parts—back, torso, arms, legs—with the "suntan" oil, then ask your partner to roll over so you can do the same thing to his or her front.

Ready to take things a step further? Guys, run your hands down the center of your partner's torso, including the area between the breasts. Encourage her to "sunbathe" topless before using circular motions to gently knead her breasts and running your fingers up and down the sides, away from the nipples and back again. Now slip your fingers under those bikini bottoms to give your partner's genitals some much-needed attention. But don't rush things: You need "sun protection," too! Now it's your turn for a massage. When you're done, dim the lights and imagine making love on the beach at night—without that pesky sand.

European Staycation

Economic woes have put a European tour out of reach for many people lately. Fortunately, you can enjoy a little Continental flavor without leaving the comfort of your hometown.

SET THE SCENE: Europe is all about historic places, artistic endeavors, stunning scenery, and scrumptious cuisine. Europeans also tend to have more relaxed attitudes toward nudity and sexuality, which makes this staycation a perfect opportunity for increasing intimacy. Remembering these themes, fill your day or week with activities meant to exude a European atmosphere: Visit a museum or two, flirting all the way. Make eyes at each other over a cup of cappuccino at your local café. Neck during a foreign film or art house movie. Indulge in a good bottle of wine; a French, Italian, or Spanish meal; and some chocolate. Hold hands in public and steal a kiss (or two, or ten).

THE PLAN: Play off of the uninhibited European point of view with a playful fashion show that will boost your body image and get your partner's motor running. Head to the closest lingerie chain store, choose some outfits, and try them on for your partner (see "Fashion Show" on page 169 for more details). Whether or not you purchase anything, you'll want to head straight to the bedroom when you get home!

Adventure Staycation

Climbing Mount Everest or swimming with great white sharks off the coast of South Africa aren't for everyone, but the sexy surge of adrenaline that adventure vacations provide can be recaptured at home for even the most skittish of couples.

SET THE SCENE: The goal of this staycation is to get your heart racing and your blood pumping outside of bed, and then translate those physical changes to what goes on between your sheets. Research suggests that a little danger can boost sexual attraction, and unpredictability goes a long way. It spikes the brain's natural amphetamines, dopamine and norepinephrine, which play a big role in sexual arousal. So get out there and shake things up by trying something new: Think of an activity that will be fresh and exciting for both of you (and maybe even a little bit scary). It could be as adventurous as white-water rafting or as seemingly mundane as singing karaoke. The point is simply to test both of your limits. Try one new activity if you've only got a day off; if you're on a longer vacation, take lessons or ramp up the excitement with a new challenge every day.

THE PLAN: Keep your adrenaline pumping at night with some activities that more obviously connect unpredictability, risk, and hot sex. What you do, of course, depends on your comfort level. While some couples might enjoy experimenting with handcuffs or other restraints, that might be too racy for others. We like the idea of a little sexy hide-and-seek: Turn off all the lights and watch a scary, but not gory, movie together. When the movie ends, engage each other in a playful game of hide-and-seek in the dark, but raise the stakes: If you get caught, you must submit to your partner's wishes.

You also might try introducing a little sensory deprivation into your bedroom routine: Place a blindfold or sleep mask over your partner's eyes and keep him guessing. Not only will he be unable to control the pace of the sex play, or the areas you choose to touch, but he won't see any of it coming. Guys, you can boost the drama even more by massaging a few drops of a female arousal gel around your partner's clitoris to heighten her arousal, sexual pleasure, and sensitivity even further.

part six

·

from
NO GO

to
THE BIG O

for both men and women alike, an orgasm (or, if you're lucky, several) tends to be the big payoff of a successful sex session. It's a stamp of approval for your partner that you enjoyed yourself in bed. But as we've discussed earlier in this book, a woman's ability to let go and climax isn't always as cut and dried as it is for guys. Men have what's called a point of ejaculatory inevitability, after which they're going to have an orgasm no matter what happens. Women don't have such a point of no return: They can "lose" an orgasm even as it's happening, particularly if they are stressed or distracted. At the same time, orgasms tend to last longer for women than for men, and with practice, you may be able to achieve multiple orgasms—or even have one just by thinking about it (see "All in Your Head" on page 152).

How you feel about your own experiences with orgasm is very individual. Some women are disappointed or frustrated if sex doesn't end in orgasm. Others find that the intimacy and connection of sex are just as enjoyable and satisfying as an orgasm. Still others may not recognize that they've had an orgasm—after all, not everybody who climaxes has a moaning, screaming, over-the-top "I'll have what she's having" experience. Roughly a third of women can't climax during sex, and about 10 percent of women have never had an orgasm at all.

To understand what you might be missing—and how to achieve it—it helps to know what we mean by *orgasm*. The term can describe a whole range of experiences, but technically, it refers to a series of involuntary muscle contractions (typically ranging between three and fifteen, at 0.8-second intervals) in the vagina, anus, and sometimes uterus. Those words hardly describe the actual *experience* of orgasm, though. When asked to describe it, most women say an orgasm begins with a feeling of tingling and warmth in their genitals, the result of masturbation, sex play with a partner, or simply fantasizing. Those sensations soon expand in waves to the lower abdominal area and other parts of the body, kind of like a physical version of a kaleidoscope. The pelvic floor muscles contract, and heart rate, breathing, and body temperature all increase until the moment of orgasmic release, when they start to return to normal.

You may have heard that there are different types of orgasms. That idea was first popularized by Sigmund Freud (yup, him again), who believed that there were two types of female orgasm: clitoral and vaginal. Although he presented little to no evidence supporting his theory, Freud claimed that so-called clitoral orgasms were a purely adolescent phenomenon, and that "mature" women should be able to have vaginal orgasms without any clitoral stimulation. Yet as we now know, about 30 percent of women require some sort of clitoral stimulation to climax. Talk about giving a third of the female population an inferiority complex!

Since then, some experts have theorized that there may be three types of orgasms, depending on where a woman is stimulated: clitoral, vaginal, and

POP QUIZ

According to the recently released National Survey of Sexual Health and Behavior, what percentage of women were "satisfied" the last time they had some nooky with their partner?

(A) 5 percent   **(B)** 23 percent   **(C)** 64 percent   **(D)** 92 percent

Answer: (C) 64 percent. What's interesting about this statistic is that while only 64 percent of women said they were satisfied, 85 percent of men said they thought their partners were satisfied. Sounds like some faking going on there, ladies!

"blended" (a combination of the two). Yet more recent evidence supports what noted sex researcher Alfred Kinsey posited in the 1950s: There is only one type of female orgasm. While it's true that stimulating different areas of a woman's body (vagina, clitoris, anus, and any number of other less-obvious erogenous zones) can lead to an orgasm, this doesn't mean that these areas and kinds of stimulation trigger different types of climax. Simply put, an orgasm is an orgasm is an orgasm.

BENEFITS OF THE BIG O

Orgasms sure feel good, but did you know that they can be good for you, too? Check out this list of ways in which the Big O can help you stay healthy:

- **Tension tamer.** Even though your heart rate and breathing spike and your muscles contract during an orgasm, they later slow, putting you into a state of relaxation. That's accompanied by the release of feel-good chemicals called endorphins, which act like natural sedatives, making you sleepy.

- **Pain reliever.** Those endorphins, as well as oxytocin (that's the cuddle hormone, remember?), also increase your tolerance to pain—by up to 70 percent, according to some studies.

- **Better body.** While it's no replacement for a healthy diet and regular exercise, orgasms may help you manage your weight: They trigger the release of phenetylamine, a natural appetite suppressant, and burn about two hundred calories after thirty minutes of sex—twice what you'd burn through sex without a climax.

- **Use it or lose it.** Orgasms help increase lubrication, as well as blood flow to the vagina, which can prevent vaginal muscles from atrophying as you age.

o my: NEW FINDINGS ON ORGASM

If you think your own orgasm is elusive, imagine how researchers feel. For years, scientists have worked with small groups of men and women to learn the ins and outs of climax. Now we have more information about the Big O, thanks to a recent large survey conducted by the experts at Good in Bed. And it's filled with both good and not-so-good news. For example, while men experienced orgasm more often than women, both sexes reported enjoying equally high amounts of sexual pleasure. Other findings:

- The factors most likely to contribute to having an orgasm were self-confidence and a feeling of connection with one's partner.

- The factor most likely to contribute to difficulty having an orgasm was mental distraction—for both men and women.

- More than 70 percent of women said they had faked an orgasm, mainly to spare their partner's feelings. Only 12 percent had discussed faking with their partner.

- More than 30 percent of men said they had faked an orgasm, mainly to bring an end to the sexual session. Only 7 percent had discussed faking with their partner.

- Both men and women enjoy orgasm equally, but only 20 percent of women say they care about having orgasm with every sex act, while 91 percent of men say that this is important.

- Forget what the romance novels tell you: A little more than a third of men and women report having simultaneous orgasms.

- Men are significantly more likely than women to report that quality and frequency of orgasm *decreased* with age.

- Women are significantly more likely than men to report that quality and frequency of orgasm *increased* with age.

GOING ALL THE WAY

Orgasms are tricky beasts: They're the result of physical or psychological stimulation (or both), which sends nerve signals between the genitals, the brain, and the spinal cord. Each part is equally important, which is why a problem in one area can affect your ability to climax. For the 10 percent of women who have never had an orgasm, a number of factors can be in play: Any medical condition, injury, or disease that affects communication between the brain and the spinal cord can interfere with orgasmic ability. More likely, trouble climaxing can be caused by certain medications, including SSRI antidepressants. Emotional issues such as inhibition, shame, and a lack of knowledge about your body and the mechanics of sex can also play a role.

For many women, the solution to problems with achieving orgasm isn't a solution at all: They fake it. As you learned in the pop quiz at the beginning of this chapter, 85 percent of men said that their partner had experienced an orgasm during their most recent sexual event, while only 64 percent of women reported actually having had an orgasm. The implication: Lots of women are faking it—and getting away with it. And, as Meg Ryan famously demonstrated in *When Harry Met Sally,* men are easily fooled.

There's any number of reasons behind this deception. Some women fake orgasm only occasionally, as a way to end an uncomfortable, exhausting, or dull sexual experience, or to preserve their partner's feelings. For other women, though, faking orgasm is a sex-life survival strategy, adopted because they've never had an orgasm or can't reach orgasm with their partner and don't want to hurt his ego.

In both cases, a variety of factors may be responsible: You might feel rushed, stressed out, tired, or distracted, for example. Or you may not be getting adequate clitoral stimulation, which the majority of women need to climax. Or you feel so self-conscious about your inability to reach orgasm that you find yourself in a vicious cycle: You feel bad, so you fake it, which makes you feel worse, so you fake it, and so on.

So . . . are you ready to come clean? You've got a couple of options. You could 'fess up to your partner, but be careful: He's likely to feel confused, hurt, and even angry when he realizes you've been lying. It's easier to tell the truth early on in relationships, when you can blame your fakery on nerves. If you've been together for a while, though, you may be better off skirting the issue while telling him how to best please you. Suggest some of the tricks in this book to increase arousal for both of you, approaching it with a fun, relaxed attitude, not sheepishness, blame, or gloom and doom. Whatever you do, *please* stop faking it—it's a no-win situation for everyone involved.

Of course, an orgasm shouldn't be the be-all, end-all of sex. If you aren't bothered by an inability to climax, your partner shouldn't be, either. (There's nothing more exhausting than a man who refuses to "give up" until he gets you off.) Still, you may be able to increase your odds of orgasm with the tips in this chapter.

GO EXPLORING. How will you know what helps get you to orgasm without experimenting? There's no better way to do that than to get to know your body and what turns you on. That's right: masturbate! It's normal—and common: Studies suggest that up to 75 percent of women pleasure themselves, whether they're single or in a relationship. So grab some lube and some privacy, and let your fingers do the walking. Don't focus on having an orgasm—just play around and see what feels good to you. Take your time. You may not climax at all the first several times, but if you make self-pleasure a regular habit, you just might get there. In fact, research shows that women who masturbate have more intense orgasms than those who don't. Plus, masturbation increases blood flow to the genitals, which is important for good sexual function in general. Once you've learned how to get yourself off, you'll be better able to guide your partner to do the same.

GET MOVING. Regular physical activity also helps promote blood flow, and also strengthens muscles, improves mood, and boosts libido. Follow Lisa's recommendations in part 4, "Lisa's 'Get Your Sexy Back' Plan," or try a yoga class: This type of exercise has been shown to improve women's sexual function, including orgasm.

ENGAGE YOUR BRAIN. Sex researcher Alfred Kinsey found that 2 percent of women could achieve orgasm by fantasy alone. And no wonder: The brain is our biggest sex organ. So let your imagination go wild. Fantasize. Watch some porn alone or with your partner, or peruse a book of erotica (see page 203 for suggestions).

RELAX AND LET GO. Perhaps one of the reasons it's easier for many women to climax through masturbation than through partnered sex is that they're more relaxed when they're alone. Some women find that the lack of distraction or self-consciousness during masturbation leads to quick orgasms. You're not worried about the way you look or how someone else feels, so you can just chill out.

When you're in bed with your partner, though, it can be difficult to let your cares go and stay in the moment. Some women find themselves doing what's called spectatoring during sex—worrying about the sex they're having while they're having it. This means you ruminate on your own performance or how your body looks so much that you can't lose yourself to the passion and simply enjoy sex for sex's sake. Another problem: You may be so caught up in all of life's big and little stresses that you can't get out of your head. And as we mentioned earlier in this book, research suggests that relaxation is key to a woman's ability to stay aroused and to achieve orgasm.

In addition to the stress management and choreplay tips listed in part 1, try putting an actual to-do list on paper before you hit the sack so that you're not so busy mentally scheduling your life that you can't focus on more pleasurable activities between the sheets. Paying attention to your breathing also helps: We tend to hold our breath as we near climax, but taking some long, deep breaths can keep you in a state of relaxation and may even intensify your orgasm.

CHOOSE THE BEST POSITIONS. Some sexual positions are better than others for encouraging your orgasm. We like female superior (woman on top) because it allows you to control the speed and angle of the action. The coital alignment technique, or CAT, is also a great choice: In this variation on the missionary position, the man puts pressure on a woman's clitoris with his pubic bone, which allows her to grind against him. Research shows that the CAT is one of the most effective ways for women to climax during intercourse. For other orgasm-friendly intercourse options, see part 5.

ADD AN ACCESSORY. Use your hand (or his) or a toy to stimulate your clitoris before or during intercourse. Remote-control-operated bullet- or egg-shaped vibrators, vibrating sheaths that fit over your or your partner's finger, vibrating penis rings, and couples' vibrators like the We-Vibe are all good choices.

PUT THE SQUEEZE ON. Kegel exercises (described on page 149) strengthen your pelvic floor muscles, which can help increase the intensity of your orgasm and that of your partner.

BE PATIENT. Some experts estimate that it takes women an average of twenty-seven minutes to climax during sexual activity with a partner. (Most guys don't last nearly as long—about two to five minutes unless they suffer from premature or delayed ejaculation.) Accept that your sexuality is different from your partner's—and that's okay. Focus on the pleasurable feelings you're experiencing, not the goal of orgasm. Remember, it's totally fine if you're in a marathon, not a sprint.

KEEP AT IT. As with sex in general, there can be a use-it-or-lose-it aspect to orgasm. The more you contract those muscles, the easier it can be to climax the next time around. So make sex a priority in your busy schedule. And when you have a particularly mind-blowing orgasm, share that with your partner. Telling him what sends you over the edge in bed (and what could be an even bigger turn-on next time) helps him understand how to keep pleasing you.

ian says . . . WHY FAKING IS NEVER OKAY

If some experts are to be believed, men need to be better educated about female sexuality, and faking is a necessary by-product of the male ego and protecting a guy's self-esteem. Personally, I don't buy it. If a tree falls in the woods and there's no one there to hear it, does it make a sound? If a woman fakes it and her partner thinks she is actually enjoying the sex, is her dissatisfaction really heard?

Don't get me wrong: As a sex and relationships counselor I'm all for education. I do believe that men get too many of their ideas about female sexuality from porn. There's no shortage of legitimate reasons why a woman might not experience an orgasm during sex, including stress, depression, anxiety, body image, performance anxiety, and fatigue. Plus, a woman may be less likely to have orgasms early in a relationship, because her body needs time to learn to trust a new partner, and she may fake orgasm in those early days as a way to show her partner she likes him. Ideally, it's a temporary situation that doesn't become a habit.

So is faking an orgasm justified? My answer used to be "yes, on occasion." But with new research suggesting that faking has become the little white lie that's amounted to a culturally accepted form of deception—most men think their partners don't fake it, while many women admit that they have—I've changed my mind. Faking every now and then is not okay. Sure, talking about sex can be difficult. It's easier to spare your partner's feelings, especially since some men may respond defensively.

But that still doesn't justify lying. Every time a woman fakes it for a legitimate reason, she undermines that legitimacy and loses an opportunity to communicate with her partner and deepen his understanding of their relationship. And don't forget: A growing number of men are now faking orgasm, too. How would you feel if you knew your guy was faking it when you had sex? It's true that talking about sex isn't always easy. But in the end, not talking about sex is even harder.

A DIFFERENT KIND OF WORKOUT

Just as you can lift weights to strengthen your arm muscles or do crunches to work your abs, it's possible to give your pelvic muscles a workout, too. Named for the gynecologist who created them in the 1940s as a way to cure urinary incontinence, Kegel exercises can increase the muscle tone of the pelvic floor, or pubococcygeal (PC) muscles. Soon, Dr. Kegel's patients began to notice an unexpected—and very appreciated—side effect of the exercises: Not only could they control their urine better when they coughed or laughed, they also found they were having more intense orgasms.

Kegel exercises work the PC muscles, a network of muscles that extend from the pubic bone, down and around between the legs, around the anus and to the coccyx (tailbone). These are the muscles that contract to help stop urine flow and squeeze the anal sphincter closed. They're also the muscles that rhythmically contract when you have an orgasm. That helps explain why research suggests that PC muscles can improve orgasms: A 2010 study found that women whose pelvic floor muscles were stronger were more likely to have better sexual function, including arousal and orgasms.

Because no one can tell when you're exercising your PC muscles, you can do Kegels anytime, anywhere—on the way to work, during a business meeting, while you're waiting in line, at the movies. Here's how to reap the benefits of Kegels:

- Locate your PC muscles. You can do this at first by trying to stop your urine stream when you're going to the bathroom. (Don't make this a habit, though, since it can actually raise your risk of developing a urinary tract infection.) You can also find your PC muscles by inserting a finger into your vagina and squeezing, or by squeezing your anal sphincter tight and then extending this squeeze all the way forward.

extra credit: MULTIPLE ORGASMS

Multiple orgasms aren't just the stuff of romance novels. In fact, most women can experience multiple orgasms, depending on the type and pace of stimulation they receive from their partners. When it comes down to it, orgasms are just the release of sexual tension, and if all of that tension doesn't dissipate the first time around—well, you've got another opportunity (and, possibly, another and another . . .). Your second orgasm may even come more easily than your first, since blood flow to your genitals is still increased and because your body is still producing the neurotransmitters associated with sex. Unlike men, who tend to lose their erections quickly (and can't get another one for a while), it takes longer for a woman's genitals to return to "normal."

If you want to encourage multiple orgasms, take advantage of this fact. Ask your partner to keep stimulating you after your first orgasm. He should slow things down and may want to avoid touching your genitals (and your clitoris in particular) for a bit, as they can be supersensitive post-orgasm. But he can keep your arousal going by stimulating your breasts, neck, and other erogenous zones. The great thing about second orgasms is that no penis is required: If he's already climaxed, he can still bring you to another orgasm with his hands, mouth, or both. It helps, though, if he's at least waited to have his orgasm until after your first: One study conducted at the University of Wisconsin found that women who were multiorgasmic were more likely to have partners who delayed their orgasms until after the women had their first ones.

Can't get there more than once with your partner? You still may be able to enjoy more than one climax when you're on your own. Most women are able to achieve multiple orgasms with greater ease during self-pleasure. In fact, Masters and Johnson found that some women were able to reach fifty—yes, that's *five-oh*—consecutive orgasms with a vibrator. These women weren't doing anything special in order to achieve multiple orgasms; they were simply providing themselves with the focused stimulation they required. So if you've got some free time and a toy or two, give it a try. You might not reach double digits, but trying can be half the fun.

■ Isolate them. Once you've located your PC muscles, learn to isolate them from other muscle groups in the area. Make sure that your legs, buttocks, and abs are relaxed and are not moving while you're squeezing your PC muscles.

■ As with any new exercise, start off slow. Squeeze and hold for five seconds, then release and repeat again for a total of ten repetitions. Try to do Kegels at least once a day and ideally three times a day. Initially you may get tired or feel the muscle losing the squeeze, but you'll have more control as you get stronger.

■ Once you have been doing regular sets of five-second squeezes for about a month, you can try to increase the squeeze time to eight to ten seconds, repeating it for three sets of ten repetitions up to three times a day.

When you feel confident that you've increased your control over your PC muscles, you can practice the squeeze while you are masturbating or during penetration with your partner. If you toned your legs, you'd want to show them off in a short skirt, right? So why not show your partner what you've learned with a little . . . shall we say, demonstration?

Start with the usual foreplay: kissing, cuddling, groping, rubbing. When you're ready for intercourse, though, slow things down. Ask your guy to enter you slowly but refrain from thrusting. Then, start flexing your PC muscles. Chances are he'll notice the sensation and be intrigued. Keep going as he thrusts, which will increase friction and pleasure for both of you. As you feel your climax approaching, continue squeezing—the rhythmic squeezing should intensify the rhythmic contractions of your orgasm. When he's ready, you can "grab on to" his penis with your PC muscles, which should send him over the edge. Don't be surprised if he asks you later if you've been working out!

advanced practice: ALL IN YOUR HEAD

Don't you wish you could wiggle your nose à la *Bewitched* and—poof!—you'd climax? While it certainly isn't that simple, it's possible for some women to have an orgasm just by thinking about it, says Dr. Emily Nagoski. It works like this: You get aroused when your brain notices sexy stimuli (say, your partner caresses your breasts) and sends messages to your genitals that give you that nice squirmy feeling. But this process works the same even if you only *imagine* a particular body part being touched. So it makes sense that you should be able to stimulate your genitals with brainpower alone. Here's how to increase your chances:

TAKE THE TIME. Give yourself an hour or two in a relaxing, private environment where you can't be interrupted.

LET THE FANTASIES FLOW. Use your imagination to picture a sexy scenario, or read a selection of erotica until you hit on something that really turns you on. It's kind of like switching channels—flip through your mental TV listing till you find your favorite. Then imagine how it would physically feel to experience that fantasy.

GET TENSE. We know, we know: We're always saying that women need to feel *relaxed* to feel aroused. And while that's true, for this exercise we're going to ask you to cultivate some sexual tension in your body. It's the tension that you feel building in your abs, butt, thighs, and pelvic floor muscles as you approach orgasm. Do some Kegel exercises now to start generating that tension.

USE YOUR BREATH. As you approach orgasm, your diaphragm muscle tends to tense as well. This shows up in your breathing, so that you gasp as the diaphragm contacts and exhale as it relaxes. Use this knowledge to pay attention to your breathing now and allow it to change. Your arousal should increase with it.

LET IT HAPPEN. As you continue along this path, you may find yourself climaxing. Yay—you did it! If nothing happens, don't worry. While it's a fun trick (and an awfully useful way of achieving a hands-free orgasm), it's not crucial for a satisfying sex life. Either way, you just enjoyed a relaxing hour alone with your thoughts!

part seven

·

new
ADVENTURES

a dmit it: Even if you're the world's biggest comfort creature, you're probably at least a little curious about certain activities outside of your usual
bedroom routine. Maybe you're content keeping those adventures strictly in
the realm of fantasy. Or perhaps you've decided it's time to dip a toe into the
deep end and start swimming. Either way, you're not alone: From sex toys, to
bondage, to anal pleasure, many couples are open to getting naughty in bed. In
fact, results of a recent survey by Good in Bed suggest that men and women are
interested in being more sexually adventurous—and that those "kinky" behaviors can boost satisfaction for both partners.

POP QUIZ

How many positions are depicted in the original *Kama Sutra*?

(A) 64 **(B)** 82 **(C)** 101 **(D)** 120

Correct Answer: (A) 64. So many positions, so many possibilities—and yet the most popular sexual position around the world is "missionary," even though the traditional missionary
approach is less likely than other positions (like "woman on top") to lead to female orgasm.
So what's the appeal of the missionary? Probably the intense eye contact it facilitates, which
connotes lovemaking as opposed to just pure sex.

It's only natural to want to explore (or think about exploring) different activities that are out of the, um, box. And fantasizing about those possibilities can play an important role in your sex life: Whether you choose to share your fantasies, act on them, or simply keep them to yourself, sexy thoughts can increase your desire and drive your arousal. The activities outlined in this section are some of those that couples tend to fantasize about. The tips here can help you make the transition from fiction to reality—or capitalize on the fantasy for maximal pleasure with your partner without going all the way.

SOMETIMES A FANTASY

Sigmund Freud gave fantasy a bad name back in 1908 when he said, "A happy person never fantasizes, only a dissatisfied one." Well, we think Freud couldn't have been more wrong—and we've got the stats to prove it. An estimated 95 percent of men and women say they have sexual fantasies, and about 70 percent of them use those fantasies as a turn-on, either during masturbation or during sex with a partner.

The truth is, a healthy fantasy life is one key to a great sex life, even if your partner doesn't always play the leading role. Fantasy isn't the sad daydreaming of the lonely, forlorn, or frustrated in love. In fact, research shows that people with active fantasy lives are *more* sexually satisfied, *more* sexually responsive, and *more* adventurous about sex in general. Take that, Sigmund.

While a lot of fantasizing takes place while we're awake, our deepest sexual longings also find their way into our dreams. Sleep puts the brain on autopilot and allows the deeper desires inside of us to come out and play. As neuroscientist Mark Solms, a leading expert in the field of sleep research, explains, "Dreaming does for the brain what Saturday-morning cartoons do for the kids: It keeps them sufficiently entertained so that the serious players in the household can get needed recovery time. Without such diversion, the brain would be urging us up and out into the world to keep it fully engaged."

So what are most of us dreaming about? A recent study by researchers at Trent University in Peterborough, Ontario, found that intercourse is the most common sexual behavior in dreams. More than a third of participants reported having a sexual dream once a week, while a staggering 19 percent reported sex dreams up to *five* times per week! Interestingly, those who reported higher

quick study: SHAKE UP YOUR SEX LIFE

Two bridges span the Capilano River in North Vancouver, Canada. The first, just five feet wide and 450 feet long, is made from wooden planks and cable and sways in the wind some 250 feet above the water. The second bridge, in a different spot on the river, is solidly built and sits just ten feet above sea level. In 1974, two well-known psychologists, Arthur Aron and Donald Dutton, used these bridges in a two-part experiment designed to test sexual attraction.

On day one, whenever a single man walked across the shaky bridge, an attractive female psychology student would stop him halfway and ask him to take a brief survey. On day two, the same woman conducted the same routine on the sturdy bridge. In both scenarios, the young woman would hand the man her phone number and tell him that he could call her later that evening for the results.

The twist? The real study had nothing to do with the survey, but with what happened afterward. Dutton and Aron wanted to know whether the excitement of standing on the shaky bridge, compared to the safety of the solid bridge, could promote romantic attraction.

The answer, it appears, is yes. The researchers found that men on the shaky bridge were more likely than those on the sturdy bridge to call the woman later for results of the survey. Not only that, but they were also far more likely to ask her for a date, as well. There's a bio-chemical basis for this phenomenon: Unpredictability increases the brain's natural amphet-amines, dopamine and norepinephrine, which play a big role in sexual arousal. Want to create your own "shaky bridge" to amp up your sex life? Try the techniques in this section of the book.

sexual satisfaction in their relationships tended to dream more often about their partner. Seventy-two percent of participants believed their sex dreams had meaning and 49 percent gained further insight into their waking relationships, past, present, or potential.

This tells us that sexual fantasies are completely normal and also provide insight into what's going on in our waking lives. There's no need to feel guilty about your fantasy life, whether you're dreaming about someone other than your partner or you're dreaming about things you're hesitant to act out in real life. Dreams free the brain to explore secret, extraordinary realms without the obligations of everyday life, so you can basically relax and enjoy the show.

But what if you want to be a key player in that show during waking hours? While many of us are content to keep our wildest dreams to ourselves, choosing to experiment a bit is completely normal. Raising the issue with your partner, though, may not come naturally, even to thrill seekers. You might worry about being rejected, laughed at, and otherwise judged. Relax: If you're in a healthy, committed relationship, it's unlikely that your guy is going to totally shut you down. While he might not personally share your same fantasy, he'll likely be open to hearing about it. If you're too shy or embarrassed, break the ice by telling him that you had a sexy dream about him: You'll pique his curiosity and he'll probably be so intrigued that he'll want more details. Then you can incorporate aspects of your fantasy into your "dream" and see how he reacts.

Or make the process into a game similar to Two Truths and a Lie, in which players share with each other two true things they've done in the past, as well as one thing they haven't. In this case, however, you share with your partner by telling him about just one sex act you've actually experienced and two you've never tried (but might like to try). This game can help you be more open about your sexual desires, and give you fodder for spicy new bedroom activities. Once you reveal your truth, tell him what intrigues you about a certain sex act, or talk about why you've found it enjoyable in the past. Touch upon any concerns your partner has about introducing it into your sex life. The goal here is to get you talking about what you've tried and would like to try. If you both decide to act out your fantasy—or just to get a little naughtier in general—use the ideas here to get started.

ian says . . . WOMEN'S TOP FIVE FANTASIES

In *A Billion Wicked Thoughts,* a book by neuroscientists Ogi Ogas and Sai Gaddam, we learn that while men are, indeed, more visual—preferring to fantasize about what they might do to that cute blonde the next cubicle over—women prefer to fantasize about what a man might do to them. In short, they're turned on by the thought of feeling desired.

How does this desire play out in their sexual imaginings? Here are women's top five sexual fantasies, and a look at where they come from.

1. Sex with someone else. In a study published by the *Journal of Sex Research,* 80 percent of partnered women said they had fantasized about someone other than their partner during sex in the previous two months. That's likely because, while sex within the context of monogamy can be totally hot, men definitely put in extra effort when they first meet someone.

2. Being dominant in bed. While it may seem counterintuitive for a woman to want to take charge when what she's really craving is the feeling of being desired, the dominatrix scenario actually revolves around the man worshipping the woman's body and begging her for attention.

3. Exhibitionism. In this scenario, a woman not only gets to enjoy sex with her partner, but also gets to enjoy the knowledge that someone else is feeling aroused by watching her in action.

4. Being sexually ravaged. How many spicy, hot movie scenes have you enjoyed in which the man pushed the woman up against the wall, forcing a kiss upon her? The thought of a man so bursting with desire is an undeniably attractive one for women.

5. Enjoying a threesome. Being worshipped and adored by two different men can be twice as nice.

So what does all this mean about women's psychological state? In my experience working with couples, fantasies are rarely a problem. Rather, they can fuel arousal in your sex life, and are a sign of high sexual satisfaction. If you can share a sexy fantasy with your partner without feeling judged or embarrassed, the intimacy within your relationship is obviously strong. When should you worry? If you're feeling bored or upset during sex, and are using fantasy as a way of disconnecting, there could be a problem. Or if you're repeatedly fantasizing about someone inappropriate—like your brother-in-law or your best friend's partner—there may be cause for worry. In one instance, for example, I was working with a young bride-to-be who was constantly fantasizing about her brother-in-law-to-be instead of the groom. These sexual fantasies were not a sign of attraction, but were actually a sign of her intense ambivalence over her impending marriage. She ended up meeting someone else who was a much better fit, and was happier for it. The day she broke up with her intended fiancé, she also stopped fantasizing about his brother.

Otherwise, don't fear your fantasies. Enjoy them. Use them to heat things up in the bedroom. And remember: There is a clear difference between fantasy and reality. And sometimes, a wacky fantasy is just hinting at another, perfectly normal desire within you.

lisa says . . . TALKING ABOUT SEX

If you're nervous about suggesting something new (and a maybe a little kinky) to your partner, you're not alone. It can be difficult for even the most candid of us to talk about sex—whether that's with our lover, our best friend, or a total stranger. I experienced this firsthand when I wrote my first book, *Rinnavation*. In it, I briefly told the story of my sexual reawakening and shared a sex tip or two. But that wasn't so hard: It was all on paper, after all, and I was pleasantly surprised by the positive reaction I received from my readers.

Howard Stern was a whole different story. I've listened to Howard for years and he had been after me to appear on his radio show for quite a while. I can't lie: I was terrified! If you've listened to Howard, you know that he loves to talk about sex. And, as freeing as it had been for me to write about the topic, I wasn't exactly comfortable sharing intimate details of my sex life on the radio with Howard and millions of listeners.

After weighing the offer for a few years, I finally gave in. I spoke with a publicist friend who gave me some great guidance (limit the discussion about sex to my life with Harry; give Howard a few tidbits—the more you refuse to share with Howard, the more he'll hound you for details!). And you know what? The interview went smoothly, I enjoyed myself, and Howard has invited me back for several more visits. As it turned out, talking about something so private in a very public setting helped me shed my inhibitions and made me more comfortable talking about sex in general.

You may not be prepping for an interview with a "shock jock," but talking about sex with your partner can seem just as daunting, especially if you're interested in trying something new and different. Here's what Ian and I recommend:

TIME IT RIGHT. You might be worried that your partner will judge you, but the truth is that most guys are intrigued and excited to learn that their lover wants to try something new. However, the time and place to start the chat are crucial. You'll want to wait until he's relaxed and happy—not when he's rushing to work, or exhausted, or grumpy. One idea: Plan a romantic evening, share a few glasses of wine, nosh on some chocolate, and let the sexy conversation flow naturally.

KEEP THINGS POSITIVE. Present your desires in a positive light. Let your partner know that you already find your sex life so exciting that you're inspired to take it a step even further. Be sure he understands that you're already sexually satisfied and that nothing is lacking in your relationship.

FRAME IT AS A FANTASY. If you're having trouble articulating what you want to do, pose it to your partner as a fantasy. Or tell him that you had a supersexy dream about him, whether that involved tying him up, or dressing as a hot cop, or experimenting with some back-door action. Chances are, he'll want to hear more.

12

BABES IN TOYLAND

You played with toys as a kid. Why not bring that playful attitude to the bedroom as an adult? Of course, your childhood playthings were probably along the lines of Barbie dolls and Big Wheels, while the toys we're talking about here are decidedly more grown-up. From vibrators to penis rings to sexy costumes, the tips in this chapter all involve a sense of fun and play—and just might seriously turn you and your partner on.

THE BUZZ ABOUT VIBRATORS

These feel-good toys have been around since Victorian times, when physicians recommended their use to treat "female hysteria." Today, vibrators have gone cordless—and mainstream. A 2009 study published in the *Journal of Sexual Medicine* found that nearly 53 percent of women used vibrators, and that those women experienced increased sexual desire, arousal, lubrication, and orgasm. Seems like those Victorian doctors might have been on to something.

If you've never experimented with a vibrator, consider what you're missing: This toy comes in a wide range of shapes, sizes, and colors and uses vibrating sensations to stimulate body parts—nipples, clitoris, vulva, vagina, and G-spot, to name a few. And those are just *your* parts. That's right: Guys can benefit from vibrators, too! So don't just get your buzz on alone. Why not include your partner in the fun? According to a recent survey by Good in Bed, 61 percent of couples are adding vibrators and other sex toys to the mix. That makes sense, since about a third of women can't climax from intercourse alone. Even if your man can last as long he likes, that doesn't mean that you're going to have an orgasm. And most sexual positions don't provide direct clitoral stimulation, which is vital to the Big O. A vibrator helps you and your partner get at least halfway home, if not taking you all the way.

If you and your guy are interested in expanding your repertoire by using a vibrator, make the whole process sexy by shopping for one together, either online or at a store. (Specialty sex shops and online retailers such as Babeland, Good Vibrations, and Pure Romance are especially women- and couple-friendly and educate customers as well as sell products.) Or drop by your local drugstore: Brands such as Trojan now make basic vibrators and other sex toys—you'll find them right next to the condoms. Vibes are available in an array of choices, usually run on batteries, and are made from silicone, latex, plastic, vinyl, or rubber. (Some vibrators are also waterproof, but be sure to check the label before trying it out in the shower or tub!) Here are some of the most common.

- **CLITORAL.** Although most vibrators can be used to stimulate your clitoris, these are made specifically for that purpose and don't always look like your stereotypical vibe: They aren't shaped like penises and instead may resemble eggs, bullets, small flashlights ("pocket rockets"), and even back massagers. Some vibes are phallic-shaped but include a small "animal" or "tongue" at the base, which is meant to stimulate the clit. The "Rabbit" vibrator popularized by *Sex and the City* is one such toy; others may look like dolphins, cats, or bears.

- **DILDO.** A dildo is a phallic-shaped sex toy that's meant to be inserted into the vagina or anus. Add some vibrations to that sucker and you've got a dildo-type vibrator. These products typically resemble a penis (either literally or just shape-wise).

■ **EGG.** Shaped like an egg or a bullet, these vibes are meant mainly for clitoral stimulation and are usually attached by a wire or cord to a handheld control. Although their small size makes them less obtrusive, many eggs and bullets offer multispeed vibrations that can pack a wallop. And check out the Tenga egg designed specifically for men, proving that toys are made for boys, too!

■ **G-SPOT.** This type of vibrator is made to stimulate your G-spot in particular. As such, they tend to be angled or curved toward the tip and made of softer materials such as silicone or jelly. G-spot vibes can also be used to stimulate a man's prostate, if he's so inclined.

■ **PANTIES/BUTTERFLY.** Panties that contain a small vibe in the crotch area, as well as butterfly-shaped vibes that strap onto your pelvic area with a thin elastic band, can offer hands-free stimulation, which your partner controls via remote control.

■ **ANAL.** Most vibrating toys that are meant for anal use have a flared base to prevent them from slipping inside the body. Some multi-use vibes include attachments that can provide subtle anal stimulation while inserted into the vagina.

■ **COUPLES.** While you and your partner can incorporate any of the toys here into sex, some vibes are made specifically for couples. The We-Vibe, for example, is a flexible, curved vibrator that you insert into your vagina and turn on during intercourse so that it provides hands-free stimulation for both you and your guy.

Now that you've got your vibrator, we hope you'll jump right in and start experimenting together. Need ideas? Try these scenarios:

FUN FACT

The original vibrator was only the fifth domestic appliance to be electrified, after the sewing machine, fan, tea kettle, and toaster.

GO SOLO. If you've previously used a vibrator for masturbation but not with your partner, use that experience to show him what you like, then ask him if he'd like to take over. Chances are he'll want to start wielding that vibe like it's a light saber and he's a sexual Jedi master.

ADD IT TO INTERCOURSE. Try using a couple-friendly toy like the We-Vibe or use an angled or egg- or bullet-shaped vibe to stimulate yourself during sex.

GIVE HIM A BUZZ. Some men are wary of being on the receiving end of a vibrator (especially those that are phallic-shaped) because they worry what that says about their masculinity or heterosexuality. The truth is, plenty of straight guys enjoy sex toys. One hot way to make him a fan of vibrators is to use one during oral sex. Hold the vibe to the outside of your cheek while you give your guy a blow job.

FEEL HIS VIBES. This is a fun trick if you've got a bit of an exhibitionist streak: Slip on a pair of vibrating panties before heading out on date night, and hand your partner the remote. Tell him to surprise you. Then go somewhere with lots of onlookers (like a crowded bar, concert, etc.) and see what unfolds.

KEEP IN MIND: Be sure to use plenty of lube with your vibrator, especially those vibes that are inserted into the vagina or anus. Worried that you could become addicted to your vibrator? Put those concerns to rest: Yes, you can get used to needing only a few minutes to orgasm with a vibrator, so when you go try to climax without the toy you might feel as if it's taking forever. In truth, it's really just taking as long as it always did pre-vibrator.

PUT A RING ON IT

Penis rings are placed around the base of the penis, and sometimes the scrotum, to improve the quality of a man's erection. Typically made of silicone, leather, fabric, or rubber, a penis ring works by trapping blood in the shaft of the penis, giving him a harder, longer-lasting erection. Some couples use penis

lisa says . . . PARTY ON

I really kicked off my own sexual reawakening in what seemed like the most unexpected place: a party. That's where I met Lou Paget and gained a whole bag of tricks for how to please a man. Since that party almost a decade ago, a new breed of get-togethers has started to replace Tupperware parties and can help you learn about sex in a safe, female-friendly environment. A bunch of companies (which go by names like Surprise Parties, Passion Parties, and Pure Romance) now market vibrators, lube, and other goodies to women at fun, at-home cocktail parties, just like Avon, Silpada, and Pampered Chef—except these gadgets are a lot more interesting! I think these types of get-togethers are a great opportunity to have a laugh with your friends while expanding your horizons and maybe even buying a few new toys. Researchers think so, too: A recent study in the journal *Sexual Health* found that in-home sex-toy parties can educate women about different products and about sex in general. Interested in hosting or attending? Hit the Internet or ask around. The popularity of these parties means you probably already know someone who's had one.

rings to spice up their sex lives, while others use them because the male partner has erectile dysfunction, although research does not necessarily suggest this works. Guys who like penis rings say they can improve genital sensation and orgasm quality. Women who like them say they help their man last longer in bed. Some penis rings can even provide vibration and clitoral stimulation to a woman during vaginal intercourse, usually by attaching to a small bullet vibrator. Like vibrators, penis rings have now hit the mainstream and you can find them from manufacturers like Trojan, right near the condoms in many drugstores.

Keep in mind: A man shouldn't wear a penis ring for longer than thirty minutes and should definitely remove it if he starts to experience any discomfort, pain, coldness, or numbness in his genitals. He may want to trim his pubic hair before using a ring to prevent it from getting caught.

STRANGERS IN THE NIGHT

Remember playing dress-up as a kid? If you were like lots of little girls, you probably had a bag or box filled with hand-me-downs, garage sale castoffs, and old Halloween costumes at your disposal. In a matter of minutes, you could transform into a princess, a cowgirl, a gypsy . . . the possibilities were endless. And when you first met your partner, you probably enjoyed a bit of primping as well, albeit in a nice dress and heels or a piece of lingerie. Of course, we all know what happens when you're in a long-term relationship: Pretty soon the garter belts get replaced by sweatpants and you're lucky if you can wipe the baby puke or dog hair from your shirt before "date night."

Well, it's time to recapture the joy of dress-up. What better way to shake things up and incorporate a little fantasy into your sex life than through some role-playing? There are so many fun scenarios to try: doctor and nurse, French maid and hotel guest, hooker and john . . . you get the idea. (And if you need more inspiration, see "Acting Out" on page 170.) If it's been so long since you felt smokin' hot that you need to ease into things, though, try these on for size:

FASHION SHOW. This is a great place to start if you're a little nervous about playing dress-up for your partner. Grab your guy and head to the closest lingerie shop. Browse the offerings individually, pick up whatever appeals to you (don't worry about the prices right now), and reconvene at the fitting room. As you try on your selections, put on a little show for your partner and talk about which pieces look sexiest. Also consider how different types of lingerie make you feel—saucy? dominant? coy?—and how each could figure into possible role-playing scenarios later. If there's a piece that seems to blow your partner's mind, splurge on it. Or, if you're more comfortable shopping solo, browse the racks, try on a few pieces, and vamp in front of the fitting room mirror. Once again, see how each piece makes you feel, and then choose a few to bring home. Later on, surprise your man at the door—wearing nothing but your favorite purchase.

AT HIS BECK AND CALL. Even pretending to have no-strings-attached sex can make you feel freer and more willing to act out your fantasies. So why not play at being an escort and her very eager client?

Dress in an outfit that's different from your usual garb—maybe a little black dress, or a miniskirt, or a low-cut top. Give yourself a new name and new persona for the night before meeting your guy at a restaurant or bar (preferably one that's new to both of you). Catch his eye from across the room, make eye contact, strike up a getting-to-know-you conversation, and flirt like crazy. Let him buy you a drink or two.

Then, when the night is about to end, suggest that you might be willing to take things further with your man—for a price. Let him slip you a few bills and take you home. At this point, the ball is in your court. You get to decide how much it will cost your man for various sexual favors. The more he's willing to spend, the hotter you'll probably feel. And that cash? Put it in a kitty toward your next date.

lisa says... ACTING OUT

Of all the sexy scenarios in this section, the one that comes most naturally to me is role-playing. After all, Harry and I are both actors: It's our job to try on different personas. I know that pretending to be someone else isn't easy for everyone, but that doesn't mean you shouldn't give it a try. Tap into your imagination, or use one of the plot ideas in this chapter to fuel your make-believe. You can even read a book of erotic stories and act out your favorite tale with your partner.

Both in and out of bed, I find that dressing the part can really help me get in character. For sexy role-playing, I love stores like Trashy Lingerie. You can also try online shops such as 3Wishes.com, check out party outlets (even iParty now sells "sexy" adult versions of some costumes), or just peruse your own closet for ideas: A short skirt and pair of high heels are versatile enough for lots of sexy situations. Here's some inspiration to get you started:

- Nurse and patient (or doctor)
- Pirate and kidnapped maiden
- Call girl and client
- French maid and hotel guest
- Teacher and student

- Cop and criminal
- Harem girl and prince
- Football player and cheerleader
- Superhero and damsel in distress

PRINCE CHARMING. Fairy tales aren't just for kids. Several have the potential for some very adult make-believe, too. Here's how to transform some of the classics into sexy role-playing scenarios:

The Arabian Nights or *One Thousand and One Nights:* In this story, a young virgin is betrothed to a Persian king who's killed all of his previous wives. She saves her life by telling him stories every night, all of which end in cliff-hangers that keep him wanting more. So gather a selection of erotic stories and begin reading them aloud to your partner. Make a note of which story turns him on the most, then stop reading and tell him to *show* you how he would finish the story.

Goldilocks and the Three Bears: Sex up this story by trying out nooky in different spots in your home—the kitchen table, the living room floor, the couch, the shower. Even if the bed ends up being "just right" after all, at least you'll have tried something new.

Sleeping Beauty: Bring your libidos back to life by taking turns kissing each other from head to toe—lips, chest, tummy, hands, genitals, feet, you name it.

Aladdin: Skip the magic lamp, but do grant each other three sexual wishes, no questions asked. This is also a great opportunity to make some of your fantasies come true.

ILLICIT AFFAIR. The beginning of every love affair starts with butterflies, racing hearts, and a sense of intrigue. Isn't it time to recapture that feeling? No, we're certainly not asking you to cheat on your man. In fact, this experiment involves just the two of you.

Start by giving yourselves permission to be someone new. E-mail each other and arrange to meet at out-of-the-way restaurants or bars. Huddle in back-corner booths, holding hands beneath the table or playing footsie. Can't help yourselves? Hightail it to a hotel room, your car, or even a dark alley for a secret tryst. Use this exercise to remind yourselves of what it was like to first fall in love—and to reignite that passion now.

ian says . . . ARE WOMEN MORE SEXUALLY ADVENTUROUS?

Although a recent survey by Good in Bed found that nearly half of couples are bored in their relationships, my colleagues and I have also learned that just as many couples believed that trying something new in the bedroom would help get them out of their rut. Naturally, we became curious about just how crazy they were willing to get in the bedroom, so we conducted a new survey on sexual adventurousness. The findings were a mix of the logical and unexpected. Perhaps the most surprising: Women are apparently way more sexually adventurous than men.

After surveying 3,100 people, we found that women were significantly more likely than men to have engaged in a wider variety of sexually adventurous activities, such as talking dirty during sex and sharing their sexual fantasies with their partners. Do women feel pressured to play the sex kitten these days, or is there something more at work?

"I think that times have changed (and continue to change) and women are becoming more and more comfortable being sexually expressive and adventurous with their partners," says Kristen Mark, M.S., a Ph.D. candidate and survey director for Good in Bed. "Women have for so long been constructed in our society as prudes who restrict the sexual expression of their male partners, and I think this survey shows that in our sample of women, that just isn't the case."

And that's a good thing. Trying new things has long been suggested as a great way to dig oneself out of a sex slump. Why? Mixing things up can cause a spike in the levels of dopamine and norepinephrine rushing through your system, thereby making you more aroused. "Usually when you try something with a partner," says Mark, "even if you don't ever do it again, the thrill of trying something new can really rev up the satisfaction level." So what are men and women trying out in the bedroom? According to our survey:

- 89 percent of women are setting the mood with sexy lingerie
- 85 percent are having sex all over the darn place: in the kitchen . . . in the bathroom . . . on the living room floor . . .
- 83 percent of men also enjoy indulging in a change of scenery
- 63 percent of men are experimenting with dirty talk during foreplay or sex.

Not only that, but stereotypically taboo behaviors were also found to be fairly common. For example, 43 percent of respondents had engaged in anal sex. Meanwhile, a whopping 61 percent had engaged in sex with the chance of being overheard, and 57 percent had engaged in exhibitionistic behavior, such as masturbating for their partner's viewing pleasure.

Then why are these behaviors still, for the most part, considered taboo? "I just think that society as a whole is not yet willing to talk about these things openly," says Mark, "so therefore they are deemed 'taboo.' And perhaps behaviors being 'taboo' is part of the excitement of engaging in them!"

Want to suggest a new sexual behavior to your partner without sending him screaming into the night? "Bringing it up with your partner by referencing this study is a great way to break the ice," says Mark. "Perhaps pick your top three exciting behaviors from our list and present it as a sort of wish list to your partner."

Relationships aren't easy. With all of the threats to monogamy these days, couples have to get creative in order to keep their relationships strong. But there's hope. Our study found that the longer you're in a committed, long-term relationship, the more likely you are to engage in a variety of sexually adventurous activities. And the saucier you become, the more likely you are to be sexually satisfied and content in your relationship. So start cooking!

13

PUSHING YOUR BOUNDARIES

*a*re the suggestions in chapter 12 old hat to you? Are you and your partner ready to go further? If so, the scenarios here—from flaunting your exhibitionist side, to experimenting with dominance and submission, to exploring anal pleasure—can definitely help push you both past your comfort zones. While you might worry that "good girls" don't do such things, we hope you'll remember our mantra: Nothing that you and your partner both try consensually is "wrong."

CAUGHT IN THE ACT

If you've already moved sex out of the bedroom and christened the other rooms in your home, you're one step closer to taking things to another level. The idea of having sex in a public place—the urgency, the thrill of possibly being discovered—is a big turn-on for many couples: In fact, about 60 percent of men and women have gotten busy someplace where they also could get caught, according to a recent survey by Good in Bed. Sound like you? Chances are you're an exhibitionist, or at least have exhibitionistic tendencies. And who could blame you: Doing something dangerously illicit can be a lot of fun!

SUBTLE STRIPTEASE. Start things off slow by undressing for your partner only. Instead of just putting on your jammies and jumping under the covers, take your time. Do what you need to beforehand to feel sexy and confident: Shave, moisturize, don some sexy lingerie. As you undress, remember how you felt when you and your partner couldn't get enough of each other, and use that memory to embolden you. No need to break into a full-on lap dance unless you want to—just make the moment more sensual than usual. If your partner's doing the undressing, give him your full attention (hide that iPhone!) and let him know how great he looks.

TOUCHING AND WATCHING. Before you start making out in public, why not put on a little show in private? You might feel embarrassed or shy at first, but masturbating for your partner can be a huge turn-on for both of you—and it can give you a better idea of how you both like to be touched. Start with your usual types of foreplay, but forgo intercourse. Instead, take turns pleasuring yourselves while the other partner watches. Want a hand? Put his over yours so he can feel just how you touch yourself.

HIGH-TECH HOTNESS. Misbehaving politicians aside, there's nothing wrong with sending your partner a sexy message or photo *for his eyes only* (unless maybe one of you is indeed running for office). Ask his permission first, and never use work-related e-mail accounts, computers, or phones to do the deed. Other than that, enjoy: Send him a saucy note about what you've got planned for him later that night, or randomly text him a cleavage shot. If you or your partner travel a lot, take advantage of modern technology to keep the home fires burning. All you need is a webcam (most computers and some smartphones come with them), free Skype software, and some privacy. Do a sexy striptease, talk dirty, or indulge in full-on cybersex with your partner.

STRIP CLUBS. "Gentlemen's clubs" aren't just for bachelor parties—or gentlemen, for that matter. If you're comfortable with the scenario, pay a visit to a strip club with your partner. Watching beautiful, sexually free women move can be a turn-on and even inspire some postclub play for the two of you. Buy your partner a lap dance so you can truly watch how he gets aroused. It's a great, safe way to explore your voyeuristic fantasies. Bonus: You'll likely pick up some ideas for your own strip show later on!

PUTTING ON A SHOW. Of course, public sex can be a big risk that you might not feel ready to take, even if you've fantasized about it. So start slow, with a bit of frisky foreplay. The specifics of this exercise depend on your schedules, but the

SAFER SNEAKY SEX

Exhibitionism might intrigue you, but nobody wants to end up in jail or on the local news! While all exhibitionist activities carry some risk (that's the appeal, right?), some options are safer than others:

- Visit your local lover's lane or find a drive-in movie theater and have fun making out in your car.

- Leave your panties at home when you go out to dinner with your partner. No one else needs to know you're going commando—but make sure he does.

- Take a camping trip sans kids. Zip up your tent and enjoy sharing your sleeping bag with your partner.

- Explore various nooks for nooky while house-sitting for your friends and neighbors. Just make sure to clean it thoroughly if you want to maintain those friendships.

- Remember the game Seven Minutes in Heaven? Revisit that preteen make-out game as an adult and spend a few minutes fumbling around in the dark the next time you pass a janitor's broom closet.

point is to keep touching each other throughout the day. Rub your partner's neck or give him shoulder massages, or gently caress his cheek. Hold hands or put your arms around each other when you're out and about. Let your guy cop a feel at the movie theater. Go to a club and grind slowly against each other as you dance. Moves like these help build anticipation and keep your libidos buzzing. Before too long, you'll want to race home and rip off each other's clothes.

GOING ALL THE WAY. Public sex isn't for everyone, but if you're going to indulge, do so wisely: It's a fine line between cultivating a sense of danger and incurring indecent exposure charges. Public restrooms (particularly single stalls with locks), elevators without alarms, darkened and uncrowded movie theaters, and even empty department store fitting rooms all have potential. Whatever locale you choose, consider carrying a small container of lube with you, and dress for easy access—skirts and dresses are ideal. Remember to stay aware of what's going on around you—but not so aware that you can't relax and enjoy the action.

POWER PLAY

Ever considered experimenting with dominance and submission? You're not alone: According to a large recent survey by *Cosmopolitan* magazine, 79 percent of women have never handcuffed a guy in bed but would like to, while 83 percent have never been handcuffed by their partner but wanted him to do it. S&M isn't for everyone, but some light bondage can be fun if you want to fool around with power dynamics. You can submit yourself fully to your partner, or be dominant and control the pace of sex. If one role feels too challenging, switch places next time.

TEACHER'S PET. Beginners who want to dabble in a little power play can start with this scenario that centers around the classic roles of teacher and student. Be sure to dress the part: If you're the sexy professor, choose a low-cut sweater, tight pencil skirt, heels, and glasses. If you're the saucy student, opt for a short skirt, white button-down shirt, and patent leather Mary Janes. Don't forget a ruler, some erotic books, and anything else that will help fuel this fantasy.

If you're the professor, have your student read aloud from a book of erotica. If he stumbles or mispronounces a word, lean him over your desk and spank him with your ruler. If you're the student, ask your professor what you can do for extra credit and flash him your panties. Or tell him that you've been a bad girl and need detention—and then some. Let your imagination go wild.

COPS AND ROBBERS. What woman doesn't love a man in uniform? Add to that the power dynamic of cop versus criminal and you've got the makings of a superhot rendezvous. Stay in the bedroom for this scenario or, if exhibitionism excites you, stage the game in your car in your driveway or garage: Have your "cop" pull over you over for speeding and see what you can do to "get off" without a ticket. Whatever situation you choose, don't forget the handcuffs.

Beg your arresting officer to let you go, and suggest some community service that will make it worth his while. He can order you to place your hands on the wall and spread your legs so that he can pat you down. Feeling argumentative? He can cuff you and lean you over the bed or have you kneel in the backseat of your car as punishment. When he's satisfied that you've learned your lesson, he can give you a ticket that's payable by the sexy act of his choosing.

ALL TIED UP. For this scenario, you'll need comfortable leather handcuffs or under-the-bed restraints. Blindfolds can also add a bit of playfulness and intrigue to your time in the bedroom. If you're the dominant one tonight, have your partner lie spread-eagled (and naked) across the bed. Attach the cuffs to his wrists and bedposts, or run a set of restraints underneath the mattress and tie down his wrists and ankles. Now put a blindfold over his eyes so that he can't control the action or see what's coming next.

Next, start teasing him: Kiss and lick him all over, caress his chest, rub your nipples up and down his torso. Drive him wild by spending a lot of time *near* his genitals without actually touching them. When he seems to be getting hotter, straddle his head and encourage him to pleasure you with his mouth. Then switch back to touching him again, using different forms of touch but still avoiding his genitals. When neither of you can stand the teasing any longer, hop on top of him for some explosive intercourse. Next time, consider switching roles and see which you prefer.

PLAYING ROUGH. Sometimes, sex really can hurt so good: Increased arousal releases feel-good chemicals such as oxytocin into your bloodstream, which can raise your threshold for pain. Things that might previously have hurt—like a smack on the butt or a bite on the nipple—now feel awfully nice. Here's how to safely experiment with rough sex.

As with all sex play, the first step is communication. Talk to each other about what you're most curious about and would like to try. Next, choose a safe word that you can utter during sex to stop the action if you're truly uncomfortable. (Hint: Don't choose words like *stop* or *no,* which you might actually mean as encouragements at the height of passion.)

Also consider adding some new toys to your collection: Nipple clamps, whips, riding crops, and restraints can all be used on submissive partners, as can items like ice cubes and hot wax. Even the palm of your hand can deliver some deliciously painful spankings.

Now get yourselves excited with some steamy foreplay so that your arousal is heightened—otherwise, you may just feel pain, not pleasurable pain. Start experimenting with your toys: If you're using nipple clamps, you can tug on them lightly to tease your partner—just don't leave them on too long, which can make removal more painful. If you're trying out spanking, start slow and soft and build the intensity as you get used to it, alternating slaps with kisses or massages. Once you've agreed on the initial ground rules, you've got lots of options to try.

THE ABC'S OF BDSM

Whether you've indulged in a little light spanking, donned a blindfold, or tied up your partner with silk scarves, you've probably dabbled in BDSM. If you haven't, perhaps this flavor of kink brings to mind images of whips and chains. BDSM is all of these things and more—with a spectrum of activities wide enough to appeal to both a seasoned pro and a skittish novice. The basics:

B IS FOR BONDAGE. From neckties, to handcuffs, to rope, to a firm grasp, bondage is all about restraining you or your partner so that your ability to move is limited and you lose your sense of control. With this range of options, bondage is pretty common and many people have at least experimented with it.

D IS FOR DISCIPLINE. The D word is all those delicious demands a dominant partner makes of a submissive one, from spanking, to ordering oral sex, to making you beg for it.

D IS ALSO FOR DOMINANCE. In BDSM, dominance means one partner exerting control over another in bed—and bondage and discipline are two ways to accomplish that.

S IS FOR SUBMISSION. Submission goes hand-in-cuff with dominance; you can't have one without the other. In so-called D/S scenarios, one partner dominates while the other submits to that partner's whim—and loves every minute of it.

S IS ALSO FOR SADISM. Sadism means getting turned on when you inflict pain, whether that means spanking, whipping, pinching, or otherwise hurting your partner. Dominant partners usually partake in sadism, while submissive partners tend to be masochistic.

M IS FOR MASOCHISM. People who identify as masochists derive pleasure from pain. They're on the receiving end of a sadistic partner's actions, and those "bad" sensations delivered by a riding crop, nipple clamps, hot candle wax, or a well-placed slap can feel awfully good.

If you and your partner are interested in exploring some or all of these areas, remember that:

S IS ALSO FOR "SAFE WORD." If you're going to experiment with any aspect of BDSM, you and your partner need to decide on a safe word—a word that, whether you whisper or shout it, will alert your partner that things have gone past your comfort zone and you want to stop or slow down. Except, don't choose a word like *stop* (or *no* or *please,* for that matter). How many of us have moaned that at the height of passion when we really meant "Oh, yes, please continue!"? Instead, opt for something that makes it clear that you want to tone things down. Random words (say, *potato,* or *blue,* or *frog,* etc.) work best.

PLAYING IT SAFE

Perhaps no type of sexual activity requires safety instructions more than BDSM. Here are our "do's and don'ts" for having a good, safe time.

- **Do** start slow. If you or your partner is new to BDSM, you may want to begin by simply blindfolding him or allowing him to gently smack your butt with his palm.

- **Don't** restrain any body part so that it loses feeling and becomes numb. Leave at least two fingers' worth of space between the body and the binding—and *never* restrain the neck.

- **Do** choose material that won't chafe or injure the person who is being tied up.

- **Don't** leave a bound person unattended or restrain someone when either of you is intoxicated.

- **Do** take your time, teasing and taunting your partner to keep him guessing.

- **Don't** forget to mix pleasure with pain, gently massaging or stimulating your partner between spanks, for example.

- **Do** remember to choose a safe word (see main text) and use it whenever you want to stop the action.

TRYING THE "BACK DOOR"

Sex toys, role-playing, and bondage are all pretty naughty, but they're also among the first things people turn to when they're looking to experiment. Anal sex is the biggest taboo for many couples: Both men and women worry that it's messy, painful, and too kinky, and some men worry that enjoying it means they're gay. But there's no need to miss out on extra pleasure because of pre-conceived misconceptions. After all, the anus and rectum are extremely sensitive areas that have about as many nerve endings as other erogenous zones. And exploring them with your partner could be just what you need to spice up your sex life.

Whether because couples have become more open-minded or because anal pleasure has become standard fare in mainstream heterosexual porn, willingness to experiment with anal sex is on the rise. Nearly two decades ago, about 20 to 25 percent of women and men said they had engaged in anal sex. But in a 2009 survey, as many as 40 to 45 percent of women and men reported having tried it.

Intrigued by what you might be missing? Before you get started, let's address some fears about anal sex. If you're worried it will be messy, go to the bathroom a few hours beforehand and take a shower. If you're worried about pain, make sure to use lube. Unlike the vagina, the anus doesn't lubricate naturally, so it's prone to tears and other minor injuries. Choose thicker lubricants or those made specifically for anal sex.

Your most important tool: communication. Talk about what you want to happen *before* you start having sex, and keep the lines of communication throughout so that you're both aware of what the other is feeling. Here's how to increase your odds of a good time, with advice inspired by sex researcher Debby Herbenick, Ph.D., author of *The Good in Bed Guide to Anal Pleasuring*.

GO DIGITAL. Before you engage in actual intercourse, ease into things with a finger or two. Start with foreplay and build some arousal with a massage that focuses on your buttocks. This can help you relax and prepare those muscles for

DISCOVERING HIS "P-SPOT"

Back in part 5 of this book we talked about the G-spot, an area of the vaginal wall that appears to trigger intense orgasms in some women. Because just a thin wall of tissue separates the vagina and rectum, it makes sense that some women experience indirect G-spot simulation through anal play and penetration.

As with the female G-spot, many men find that stimulating the prostate gland, or "P-spot," in combination with another sexual activity can intensify an orgasm. The prostate gland sits just below the bladder and against the rectum wall. You can feel it a few inches inside the anus toward his belly. Once you've discovered it, have fun trying out different kinds of touch to see what works. If your guy is game, you can stimulate his prostate by penetrating the anus with a finger or dildo.

more action. With a lubricated finger, your partner can then begin exploring. Make things easier by pushing out with your buttocks as he pushes his finger inside. And don't feel you need to be on the receiving end: Some men find anal play pleasurable themselves, particularly if it stimulates the prostate (see "Discovering His 'P-Spot,'" above).

As he explores, he or you should keep stimulating your clitoris and labia to aid in relaxation and arousal. When you're ready, your partner can try to stimulate your G-spot or you can try to stimulate his prostate gland by pressing gently but firmly against the rectal wall. Or try thrusting in and out with several fingers to mimic the shape and motion of a penis or dildo.

ORAL OPTIONS. Also known as rimming, analingus means licking, sucking, or penetration the anus with your tongue. As with manual stimulation, you should both feel relaxed and comfortable. You can caress and kiss your partner's lower back, buttocks, and thighs before beginning to lick and kiss the anal opening.

good idea: SAFETY FIRST

As with any sexual act, anal play can spread sexually transmitted infections (STIs) including HIV, gonorrhea, syphilis, hepatitis B and C, herpes, the human papillomavirus, and chlamydia. You can limit your risk by using various barriers, such as the following:

- **Condoms.** Because rectal tissues can tear easily, infected fluids can enter the blood-stream. Used properly, condoms reduce the risk of HIV, chlamydia, and gonorrhea. Even if you're healthy and in a monogamous relationship, your guy should wear a condom to protect against bacteria that can irritate the penis.

- **Dental dams.** Unprotected oral-anal sex contact can also spread STIs, although the risk is lower. Plus bacteria or parasites in the lower gastrointestinal tract can trigger illness if it makes it into a person's mouth. You can reduce these risks by using a barrier such as a dental dam between the mouth and the anus. Originally made for use by dentists, these products are also now sold specifically for oral sex and are available in a variety of colors and flavors.

- **Gloves.** Some STIs such as herpes and genital warts can be transferred through genital contact alone, particularly if you have an open sore or cut on your finger. Gloves can protect you from these risks and, when lubricated, may even feel more comfortable.

The anus contains potentially harmful bacteria that can trigger infections if spread to the vagina. Reduce your risk with these two easy steps:

- Thoroughly clean anything that's been in the anus before it goes into the vagina. That includes toys, as well as your partner's fingers, penis, and mouth.

- Always use a fresh condom, dental dam, or glove when switching from anal to vaginal or vice versa.

TOY WITH IT. Once you feel comfortable having his fingers inside you or his mouth on you, try adding a few playthings, such as vibrators, dildos, plugs, or anal beads. But be sure that your toy is made specifically for anal play and has a flared base or handle so it doesn't get "lost" inside the rectum and necessitate an embarrassing trip to the ER. As additional safety measures, slip a condom over these toys, be sure to use a lot of lube, and clean your toys after every use.

READY FOR ACTION. Many people might assume that anal sex means intercourse, but that doesn't have to be an option at all if you'd prefer to stick with some of the other anal activities here. If you'd like to take that step, however, begin as you would with any other encounter: Kiss, enjoy some hand or oral stimulation of the genitals, or even have vaginal sex. Once you're aroused, you can move on to some of the types of anal foreplay described earlier. Then your partner can enter you—*very slowly*—and wait for your okay to start moving. When he does move, it should be gently and he should follow your lead. Common positions for anal sex include doggy style, modified missionary (with your legs up), woman on top, and reverse cowgirl. Whatever you choose, experiment, stay safe—and have fun!

ian says . . . FUN WITH FETISHES

As a sex counselor, I'm often asked by friends, acquaintances, and even strangers about the "weirdest" things my clients tell me. Confidentiality aside, I don't have many "weird" tales to share anyway. Most sexual complaints tend to be rather ordinary: sex ruts, mismatched libidos, erectile disorder and premature ejaculation in men, and orgasm problems and painful sex for women.

A much smaller percentage of people do have unusual sexual fetishes (also known as paraphilias)—most of them men. Women have their own unique turn-ons and turnoffs, too, but when it comes to having a favorite fantasy versus having an obsession in which all sexual pleasure is almost exclusively derived from a single object, body part, or sex practice, more men seem to have fetishes.

In their book *A Billion Wicked Thoughts,* neuroscientists Ogi Ogas and Sai Gaddam suggest that men are more predisposed to have fetishes because men are typically aroused by a single cue at a time—bare breasts, or long legs, or lesbian porn, for example. Women, on the other hand, require a seemingly endless number of cues for arousal—say, a man's deep voice, his muscular chest, the temperature of his bedroom, the thread count of his sheets . . . You get the idea.

Experts have long known about the existence of sexual fetishes, which could easily fill an encyclopedia with thousands, if not tens of thousands, of entries. Yet the origins of fetishes

➤

remain unclear. The American Psychiatric Association recognizes fetishes, but there's much professional disagreement on how to treat them and whether treatment can even be effective.

According to Freud, fetishes stem from a man's fear of castration or his unconscious fear of his mother's genitals, for example. Many psychologists continue to believe that some sort of "sexual imprinting" must occur in the early childhood of the fetishist for sexual excitement and the fetish object to become so intricately enmeshed.

Today, fetishes are often treated with a combination of psychoanalysis (the search for deep unconscious meaning behind a fetish), cognitive behavior therapy (in which the fetishist's thoughts are viewed as irrational ones that can be reversed with conscious mindfulness), and/or psychiatry, which seeks to alter the brain chemistry of the fetishist through drugs.

Luckily, many people who would normally be troubled by a fetish can now connect with like-minded peers through the Internet and/or can enjoy erotic stimulation (such as specialty porn) that caters to their specific interests. They may even be fortunate enough to have sexual partners who, as columnist Dan Savage says, are sexually GGG ("good, giving, and game") and are willing to accept and incorporate their partner's fetish into their sex play. One single woman I know even joked that she'd love to meet a foot fetishist: At this point in her life, a good foot massage sounded better to her than sex. So if you've got a partner who has a fetish, work together to determine how that fetish fits into your relationship: If you can have hot sex together and allow him to enjoy his fetish with or without you (through porn, for example), you'll have met this goal.

part eight

·

THE
ins and outs
OF PORN

What do you think of when you hear the word *pornography*? Dirty old men in dark theaters with sticky floors? Overly tan bimbos with enormous fake breasts? Charlie Sheen's latest round of "goddesses"? Sure, porn can be all of these things. But it can also be sensual, fun, and another useful device in your sexual tool kit when you indulge in it as a couple. At the same time, porn can be a source of problems in some relationships if one partner becomes dependent on it for stimulation.

The ubiquity of the Internet means that porn is more accessible than ever before. Just a few decades ago, if a man wanted porn, he had to make a trip to a convenience store magazine rack or the back room of his local video rental store. That meant he probably had a small stash of favorite masturbation material. These days, though, everything from amateur video clips, to the Victoria's Secret catalog, to hard-core fetish porn, is just a click away. That accessibility presents new challenges for both men and women: On one hand, it allows couples to enjoy porn together without the potential embarrassment of leaving home to shop for it. Yet the Internet has also made it easier for men to become dependent on the high levels of novelty that porn provides, leading to an increased risk of problems like delayed ejaculation.

The key, of course, is learning how to use porn wisely. It helps to know how you both define pornography. And that's not always so clear-cut. As U.S. Supreme Court Justice Potter Stewart famously said during a 1964 obscenity trial, "I know it when I see it." In general, though, porn is the portrayal of explicit sexual subject matter for the purpose of arousal. In other words, it's sexual stuff that's meant to turn people on. That can mean videos and DVDs, books, magazines, Web-based images, and even artwork and video games. Think porn is too "dirty" for you? We encourage you to start exploring all the different varieties and genres before writing it off. Who knows? You might just find a favorite new pastime.

LISA'S STORY: THE NAKED TRUTH

I have a confession to make: I enjoy porn. I just took the deepest breath while writing that. The truth is, it's difficult to admit without worrying that I'll be judged. I know that not every woman feels comfortable looking at or watching porn. In fact, on the occasions I've talked to my girlfriends about pornography, I've mostly been met with looks of horror and disgust. "Eww" is the most common reaction, followed closely by, "I just don't do that kind of thing." And, really, who could blame them for feeling that way? As women, we're conditioned to believe that only "bad girls" make porn—and only "bad girls" watch it.

I used to feel the same way. But once I found myself in a safe, loving, relationship with Harry, I starting becoming more willing to experiment and explore. I've said it before and it bears repeating: I firmly believe that nothing sexual that a couple does consensually and safely is "wrong." While porn certainly isn't the centerpiece of our love life, it definitely plays an occasional role. Like most long-term couples, Harry and I sometimes need a little push in the arousal department, and porn can provide that spark for us.

Don't get me wrong: I'm not a fan of all porn. Anything violent or degrading, for example, is strictly off-limits. But I've found that some films, particularly those produced by more female-friendly companies such as Vivid, can be both visually appealing and sexually arousing. If you haven't dabbled in porn, I encourage you and your partner to give it a shot. Ask him what he likes and shop together for products that appeal to both of you. Then cozy up together on the couch or in bed for a little late-night film festival!

14

WHY PORN IS
SO POPULAR

What is it about porn that's just so darn appealing to men? Well, first of all, men are very visual creatures. (Don't believe us? Just put on a negligee or take a lap around your living room naked and see what happens.) A guy sees something sexy, neurons start firing, blood starts rushing to his genitals, and bang—he's ready for action. That's why Viagra has proven so successful with men, but why female Viagra has basically been a bust. Men respond much more readily to external visual triggers whereas women can see something sexy, recognize it as sexy, but not necessarily want to have sex. That's not to say that women don't respond to visual stimulation, either, or that that stimulation doesn't lead to genital arousal—but that arousal doesn't always trigger desire in women the way it does in men.

In other words, although it certainly doesn't hurt, women generally require more than a clip of Jon Hamm on *Mad Men* to get all hot and bothered. But show a guy Don Draper's curvy redheaded colleague, Joan (played by the gorgeous Christina Hendricks), and he's likely already fantasizing about bending her over a leather Eames chair.

Then there's the novelty aspect of porn. Of course, it's often unrealistic—how often do *you* greet the cable guy with a blow job or indulge in anal sex on the hood of a Ferrari?—but that's also what makes it so hot. Porn allows us to let go and vicariously live out our fantasies, especially those that we'd never dare try in real life. There's no such thing as boring, routine sex in porn: Every action is exciting, different, risky, and over-the-top sexual.

Men may still be the primary consumers of porn, but they're not the only ones who enjoy it. In fact, not only are women increasingly comfortable and confident in asserting their opinions on the subject, but they're also enjoying porn themselves. According to a recent poll by *Glamour* magazine, 87 percent of women ages twenty-five to thirty-nine say they enjoy porn as part of a healthy sexual lifestyle. In Ian's experience, more women are using porn to satisfy a general curiosity about sex overall, to get themselves in the mood for sex or to enjoy their sexuality on their own, and to learn new sexual techniques or to explore sexually adventurous situations.

That's a sea change because, as Lisa points out, generations of women have been told that porn is evil; that it exploits, objectifies, and degrades women; and that a woman who enjoys porn is a betrayer of all women. Plus, many women have contended that porn was never really created with female customers in mind and was instead designed to appeal to men and lacked elements that were more organic to female sexuality, such as foreplay, intimacy, and erotic storylines.

Today, however, there are many porn sites geared toward women. There's even a regular Feminist Porn Awards that recognizes erotic entertainment that is smart, sexy, and appreciates women as viewers. Combine this new recognition

FUN FACT

Recently, a researcher from the University of Montreal set out to study whether pornography had an impact on guys' sex lives. He searched for men in their twenties who'd never looked at porn. Guess what? He couldn't find a single one.

of a female audience with the rapid proliferation of easily accessible Internet porn, and it only makes sense that more women are viewing porn, too.

Women may even be able to view porn with less guilt. In Ian's experience, women tend to worry a lot more about their man's porn habits and what it means to their relationship, whereas many of the men he's spoken with tend to be intrigued by the idea of women and porn—especially since women are much more likely to enjoy porn that does not directly reflect their sexual orientation. This suggests that the enormous variety of material offered by the Internet could actually end up playing more to the spectrum of female desire than to male desire in the long run.

ALL PORN, ALL THE TIME

First came the Internet. Then came broadband. And pretty soon, what was once relegated to "adults only" theaters, bookstores, and video rental shops was available to everyone with just a few clicks of a mouse. The numbers are staggering, if unsurprising: In 2007, about a quarter of all Internet searches were related to pornography. By 2010, more than a quarter of U.S. Internet users—that's sixty million people, or about one-fifth of all Americans—had searched for porn. Factor in the increasing popularity of smartphones and iPads, and you've got a situation in which anyone can access porn, anytime and anywhere.

This extreme accessibility and instant gratification hasn't just affected our browsing histories and our wallets (after all, much Internet porn is free). For better or worse, it's shifted the whole playing field of sexual relationships, from the frequency with which people—mostly men—masturbate, to the way couples connect, to the way we view our bodies and those of our partners. Frustrating? Oh, yeah. But like it or not, porn is here to stay. It's up to you and your partner to make it work for you.

15

THE GOOD, THE BAD, AND THE UGLY

When it comes to pornography, there's a fine line between pleasurable and problematic. First, the good news: Porn and masturbation usually go hand in, er, hand. And there's nothing wrong with masturbation. In fact, it's perfectly healthy—and not just a last resort for the lonely. When couples are in good relationships, they actually tend to masturbate *more* than when they're not. When people stop masturbating, it's generally a bad sign: It can mean they're depressed or have a health problem. There's nothing wrong with porn in a healthy relationship. It's just another form of masturbation material: a visual fantasy.

Porn can also be a great way to explore forbidden taboos. Fantasies are fantasies for a reason—because they're not real. So if you're interested in fetish porn, bondage, domination, or anything, it's a chance to explore things that you normally don't get to explore. There usually isn't always a direct relationship between the stuff we look at and the stuff we actually want to try, so porn can be a safe way to vicariously experience those acts.

Porn can also teach us about our unique turn-ons and turnoffs: You may find that domination really appeals to you, for example, and you'd like to share a fantasy about it with your partner, or even experiment with it. Porn is generally a pretty extreme version of a fantasy, which is why it can be so threatening to a partner, but there are usually ways to dip a toe into the water without jumping into the deep end. For example, bondage porn often involves sex slaves in extreme situations, but that doesn't mean there isn't a way to explore some light bondage within a trusting relationship.

Sometimes porn can even tell you something that you didn't know about yourself or help you identify an emotional need that isn't being met. Being tied and bound can represent a need to relinquish control, for example. There isn't a precise science to this, just the idea that our fantasies—the ones we spontaneously imagine in our heads, as well as the ones we seek out via porn—can tell us something about our unmet emotional needs.

THE TROUBLE WITH PORN

Those are the many positive effects of porn, but we'd be lying if we said there weren't some downsides, too. Antipornography crusaders have tended to focus on the more dramatic consequences of porn: They claim that it demeans women and promotes rape and other violent crimes. However, evidence that links pornography to crime is mixed at best and most research on the subject has been inconclusive.

Porn's actual effects are certainly subtler but still troubling. They can range from mild annoyances to serious dependency—and can have a very real impact on your relationship. Maybe the problem starts small: A guy has easy access to his computer and masturbates to porn once a day, simply because it's there. But then he's a little less motivated to have sex with his partner. It reduces his incentive, because he's already gotten off. These men are often older or have been in long-term relationships. They still love their partners, and if they hadn't masturbated they might be more inclined to engage their partners and pursue real sex. Instead, they squander their mojo with porn.

Pornography can also be a crutch for some guys: They may feel that masturbating to porn is easier than having sex. Less work, less hassle—so they get lazy about their relationship and don't work as hard to have sex. These men stop being as romantic or as focused on their partners, and their relationship, in and out of the bedroom, starts to suffer.

Porn starts to become a bigger problem when a man is tuned out of his relationship and uses masturbation to avoid sex, or as a substitute for sex. In the end, you have to have the kind of relationship that inspires you to *want* to have sex with your partner, so if you're angry at your partner, or not working hard to attract your partner anymore, porn can become a substitute. This is also a common issue with new dads: After having a baby, they're not touching their partner for a few months, so they start touching themselves and get into a pattern. And a lot of moms are so tired, and channeling so much energy into the baby, they're all too happy to turn a blind eye to their husband's porn use.

Porn can also become a problem for single men who are not dating and who masturbate heavily. That's fine, except when those guys start to withdraw and pull back from women, and porn starts to reinforce their disconnection. The same thing happens with guys who avoid intimacy because they suffer from a sexual problem like premature ejaculation or erectile dysfunction. For these men, porn is part of a cycle of withdrawal and depression.

YOUR BRAIN ON PORN

When you think of porn's effects on your various body parts, your brain probably isn't the first organ that springs to mind. But the nervous system actually plays a big role in sexual arousal, and porn is no different. Remember dopamine, that feel-good neurotransmitter that fans the flames of lust? The same chemical that drives that can't-keep-your-hands-off-each-other feeling in new relationships also activates the brain's pleasure centers when we look at pornography. Dopamine is also associated with the reward system of the brain, so that when we engage in something pleasurable—food, drugs, and, yes, sex—those reward centers light up and more dopamine is released. You can see how easy it is to become addicted to, or at least dependent on, whatever pleasurable trigger stimulates this process.

Some researchers also believe that a protein called delta FosB, which has been shown to accumulate in the neurons of rats when they engage in potentially addictive behavior, such as using drugs, consuming sugar, and even running, may spur porn dependency. Over time, enough delta FosB may build up that it changes brain chemistry. Although it's a long way from rats to humans, these scientists theorize that porn could have similar effects on men, reinforcing new connections between neurons every time they see pornographic images until they begin to associate porn with pleasure and vice versa.

Whether or not you choose to believe these theories, it's clear that porn use can indeed change the way sexual partners interact with each other. We think *addiction* is a pretty strong word, but it is possible to become dependent on it. In addition to the scenarios described earlier, porn can mess with a guy's skills when he does have sex. With so many varieties of porn literally at their fingertips, men can get in the habit of having a steady flow of sexual novelty and intense visual stimulation. As singer John Mayer confessed in an interview with *Playboy,* "You wake up in the morning, open a thumbnail page, and it leads to a Pandora's box of visuals. There have probably been days when I saw three hundred vaginas before I got out of bed."

As a result, many men have lost touch with their erotic memories and have become dependent on this intense and instant visual stimulus. Instead of using their creative mind for sexual fantasies, they use a variety of images to jump-start their arousal. That means that they can have a more difficult time reaching peak levels of sexual arousal with their real-world partners. They may get an erection, but they're mentally not at peak arousal. They're unable to focus fully on the sex they're having and have become habituated to high levels of visual stimulation.

Porn use (and in turn, frequent masturbation) can also affect a guy's ability to climax with a partner. When a man masturbates, he often applies significantly

higher levels of pressure and friction than real intercourse provides. If he masturbates frequently, he may get used to a different kind of physical sensation,
which only his hand can provide. That's called an "idiosyncratic masturbatory
style." As a result, a lot of men can only get past the point of no return via oral
sex, or manual stimulation (usually their own), but can't get there during sex
anymore, a condition called delayed ejaculation (DE). Although DE can have
other causes, a major trigger for the problem is frequent masturbation and porn
use. We'll talk more about DE in part 10 of this book.

WHEN PORN BECOMES A PROBLEM

An increasing number of women may be more open to porn than in the past,
but that doesn't mean they're thrilled to discover their guy's secret stash or
extensive Internet browsing history. Find us a woman who feels great about
herself and her sex life after catching her partner surreptitiously downloading
XTube videos or perusing the latest issue of *Barely Legal*—we're pretty sure
she doesn't exist (except maybe in porn!). Pornography can make even the
most sexually confident woman question her attractiveness, especially if her
guy is spending more time getting graphic with his graphics than he is with
her. If that's happened to you, you've probably found yourself wondering if
you're not exciting enough for him or whether he really wants to be with a
woman who looks and acts like a porn star. Before you start feeling too hurt
or betrayed, though, consider this: His porn use likely has very little to with
you. *Really.*

It helps to understand a bit about men in general. Porn is seemingly everywhere, and it's nearly impossible to get online these days without encounter-
ing the opportunity to get off. Often it starts off innocently: A man could be
surfing the Web in search of the latest baseball scores, when up pops an ad for
the *Sports Illustrated* issue. Guy. Bikini-clad babe. You know how it's going

to end up. And that's fine. For many guys, porn is basically a thirty-second spa day, complete with happy ending. It feels good, relieves stress, and functions as a quick little treat—kind of like scarfing down a bag of Gummi Bears in the middle of the day. It doesn't mean they're not interested in having "a real meal" with the woman they love, but sometimes they're in the mood for a snack. No big deal.

Of course, things aren't always so simple. If you suspect your guy might have a problem with porn—he's never "in the mood" for sex, yet you catch him minimizing his Internet windows every time you walk by, or he can't climax without finishing off with his hand—it's time to have a talk. Don't be confrontational. Instead, approach the situation constructively. It's too easy to let yourself get hijacked by anxiety, fear, panic, and uncertainty. And try not to take it personally. Instead, view the issue as an opportunity to have an honest talk about sex—and a chance to deepen your shared intimacy. First, ask yourself these questions:

1. Has he lost his mojo? Is he less interested, or no longer interested, in sex? He may well be squandering sexual resources that should be reserved for his sex life with you.

2. Does he seem detached and disconnected during sex? Some men become so habituated to the intense visual stimulation of porn that they're no longer able to focus on the sex they're having.

3. Is it taking him longer to reach orgasm, or is he not reaching it at all? Some men end up developing a masturbation style that is quite different (in terms of pressure and friction) from what it feels like to have sex with a person.

4. What's your overall relationship status? Are you generally tuned in and turned on, or tuned out and turned off?

During your conversation, ask your guy for honest answers to the following, which can be warning signs of porn dependency:

1. Does he always masturbate via porn? Has he become reliant on external visual stimulation as opposed to his own imagination or memories?

2. Does he use porn because he's sexually frustrated in your relationship?

3. Is his use of porn tapping him out erotically, leaving little to nothing for you?

4. Is he spending too much money on porn sites?

5. Is his use of porn getting in the way of work or other day-to-day responsibilities?

6. Does he think about pornographic images/scenes when he's actually having sex?

7. Does he feel pressure to perform like a porn star?

8. Does he judge your sexual performance based on images from porn?

9. Is his use of porn an entirely solo activity, or does he share it with you?

10. Is he hiding his use of porn from you?

If your guy has developed a dependency on Internet porn, it's important to unplug the computer and go cold turkey. But that doesn't mean that he has to stop thinking about sex altogether. Instead, use this time as a way to amp up your sex life with *each other*. Remember when porn wasn't so easily accessible to you and your partner? Sure, guys turned to magazines or videos. But they also relied on their imaginations and their erotic memories. Even sexy books and artwork force you to use some creative thinking. So try the following tips, together, to let your erotic imaginations flourish, and see where they take you.

SEXY PORN ALTERNATIVES

Whether you're concerned about your guy's porn habit or just want to spice up your sex life, these ideas can help.

TAKE A WALK DOWN MEMORY LANE. Think back to the beginning of your relationship, when sex wasn't necessarily guaranteed. When you did get physical with your partner, you probably spent some serious time daydreaming about the encounter afterward: the way he touched your body, the look in his eyes when he climaxed, the exciting new moves you tried with him. You could get yourself all hot and bothered just reliving these details. And it's not much different for men. Sure, your guy might rely on online images of busty babes to get off

---

ian says . . . GOOD (IN BED) READS:

I can't believe how few couples read erotica together. That was a big part of my courtship with my wife, Lisa. Once upon a time, back before we had kids, our life revolved around sex—and that including reading erotica aloud to each other. Sounds quaint in our age of porn, but erotica is great because, in the spirit of reading and not just watching, it really gets the imagination going and the neurons firing. So I'd like to make a plea for a return to erotica. Some of my old favorites include:

A. *The Story of O,* by Pauline Réage

B. *Emmanuelle,* by Emmanuelle Arsan

C. *Delta of Venus,* by Anaïs Nin

D. *A Sport and a Pastime,* by James Salter

E. *The White Hotel,* by D. M. Thomas

F. *Quiet Days in Clichy,* by Henry Miller

On the contemporary front, I love the anthologies that are published by Cleis Press and edited by Rachel Kramer Bussel.

now—but you've undoubtedly starred in his fantasies, too. So put yourselves back in center stage by settling in for a little reminiscing. Talk about specific instances that were particularly memorable and how they made you feel: Maybe you made passionate love while caught in a thunderstorm, or you snuck onto a golf course for some midnight nooky, or you experimented with sex toys for the first time. Use the little details of these memories to help you spark new ones.

SHARE A STORY. Just like pornographic pictures and films, "adult" literature is made to turn us on. The difference? Books tend to require us to at least partly use our imaginations. There's something for everyone, including short stories, poems, novels, memoirs, and even sexual manuals. Of course, you can (and maybe already do) enjoy sexy stories on your own. But we're all for sharing the literary love, especially when you're trying to take the focus off of visual porn. Cuddle up and read together. Before you know it, you just might find your minds wandering—and your hands straying.

APPRECIATE ART. Yes, art is visual. But we think there's a big difference between the blow-by-blow (job) depictions of graphic sex found in films and online and a static piece of erotic art that leaves something to your imagination. Spend some time with your partner perusing the wide range of sexy images out there. From suggestive nudes like Giorgione da Castlefrano's *Reclining Venus* and Pompeian drawings of couples practicing cunnilingus, to early black-and-white snapshots of saucy acts and more recent offerings from Robert Mapplethorpe and even Georgia O'Keeffe, you've got a lot to choose from. Talk about why a particular piece turns you on: Good art is a conversation starter—and this conversation could take you and your partner to some pretty sensual places.

16

INDULGING
TOGETHER

Too much porn may be a problem, but when you use it wisely, it can be a boon to your relationship. Some women are understandably bothered when their partners look at porn in secret, but they're often more than willing to explore it together. When you and your partner share porn, it can make you even more excited about sex with each other and be a strong bonding experience. Once couples start discussing porn, it's a stimulus to their relationship—to sharing fantasies, talking about likes and dislikes, and more. Looking at porn together can be a powerful way to spice up your love life and connect on a whole new level.

Shop together for movies that appeal to you both. Porn is no longer the stuff of dark, dreary theaters or closeted back rooms of video rental stores. Specialty shops such as Amazing, Good Vibrations, and Babeland are aimed at men and women alike, with the goal of making shopping a friendly, sex-positive experience. You can also surf the Web for online stores, or download movies directly (beware of computer viruses!). If you're new to porn, ask your guy what he recommends, or consult books and websites that review erotic films (see "Favorite Flicks" on page 206).

Once you've both decided on a movie, it's time to sit back and enjoy the show. Dim the lights and get cozy in the den or bedroom. A few ground rules:

FAVORITE FLICKS

With the sheer amount of porn—from movies, to books, to magazines, to websites, and more—available these days, choosing something that appeals to both you and your partner can be daunting. Make your search a little simpler by checking these resources for suggestions:

- **Hotmoviesforher.com.** This female-friendly site features porn reviews by and for women; once you find something you like, you can pay by the minute to stream it on your computer.

- *The Smart Girl's Guide to Porn.* In this book, sex educator Violet Blue offers helpful advice for incorporating porn into your sex life, along with recommendations for finding porn you enjoy.

- **Goodvibrations.com.** Offers a carefully curated selection of adult movies, with categories ranging from "Feminist Porn" to "Hot with No Plot." The site also includes free guides to choosing porn. Babeland.com has a similar library of DVDs for purchase, including those directed by women.

- **Candida Royalle's Femme Production**s is dedicated to creating porn that focuses on female pleasure, and gives couples positive sexual role modeling.

You might feel silly or nervous and find yourself giggling or mocking the on-screen action. That's totally understandable. But keep the running commentary to a minimum: Nothing kills the moment faster than one partner dissecting what's happening, while the other is trying to get turned on—unless, of course, you're suggesting how you and your partner might replicate a similar act your-selves!

So what *should* you do? Relax. Pay attention to the way you feel when you watch—your emotions, your body, everything. Notice which scenes arouse you and your partner the most. If you're feeling adventurous, start acting out what you see on the screen. No, we're not suggesting that you grab your nurse's uniform and start playing doctor (although you should certainly file that scenario away for future role-playing reference). But if you notice that your guy is getting turned on by an on-screen blow job, for example, by all means offer him a little oral pleasure while he watches. Later, talk about which scenes appealed to you each. You'll get ideas for your next video choice—and inspiration for some new bedroom activities, too.

PORN, STARRING . . . YOU!

Is one of your gripes about porn that you find the actors and actresses a bit . . . unrealistic? Does it bother you that your guy is getting off to photos or videos of other women? While porn often has little to do with what's going on in a man's real-life relationship, why not give him a little inspiration that puts *you* back in focus?

Remember that episode of *Sex and the City* where Charlotte, troubled by her husband's use of *Juggs* as masturbation material, replaced the models' faces with photos of her own? These next two exercises are somewhat in that spirit, but instead of being sneaky, you'll engage your partner to make the process itself sexy and fun.

STRIKE A POSE. For this activity, you'll need a camera, preferably digital—who wants the embarrassment of developing these pics at the local photo lab or accidentally "sexting" your friends photos from your phone? Choose a location: The bedroom is always a good choice, particularly if you add some nice throw pillows, blankets, and mood lighting. Next, get dressed up in something that makes you feel sexy, whether that's a piece of classy lingerie, crotchless panties, or your birthday suit. Now, start posing. Unless you're used to this sort of thing, you're probably going to feel a tad uncomfortable and self-conscious. Work through it! Channel your inner Heidi Klum (or Betty Page, or Paris Hilton, or Jenna Jameson . . .). Stand with a hand on your hip, or stretch out on the bed. Props are good too: "Read" a book wearing just your sexy librarian glasses and a smile. Touch yourself with a toy. Blow a kiss at your cameraman. All the while, pay attention to the way you feel. Are you shedding your inhibitions along with your clothes? If you'd like a few snaps of your guy, switch places with him and direct his sexy photo shoot. When you're done, look at the pictures together and decide which ones appeal to you most. You could print out a few to save for your partner (or yourself). Or, if you're worried about the photos falling into the wrong hands, simply delete them. Remember, this activity is more about the journey than the destination.

FILM FEST. Has your "movie night" inspired you and your man to try shooting your own flirty flick? As with the erotic photography exercise, you may initially feel foolish, but putting yourself in the spotlight can be a big ego boost in the

good idea: FILM FEST

Don't quite feel comfortable sharing porn with your partner just yet? Ease into the hard-core stuff by indulging in a sexy R-rated flick together first. Some of our favorites:

- *9½ Weeks*
- *Basic Instinct*
- *The Big Easy*
- *Body Heat*
- *Eyes Wide Shut*
- *Henry and June*
- *Last Tango in Paris*

- *Like Water for Chocolate*
- *Lust, Caution*
- *Secretary*
- *Sex, Lies, and Videotape*
- *Unfaithful*
- *Y Tu Mamá También*

long run. So set up a camcorder or other recording device (such as a Flip) in your bedroom, living room, or otherwise private and kid-free space. Set it down on the dresser or other level surface, or use a tripod if you have one. Experiment with lighting (if you're making a simple sex tape) and props (if you're aiming for a role-playing or plot-heavy scenario). Shop your closet for a getup that makes you feel hot, whether it's a sassy schoolgirl outfit, a role-playing costume, or a silky bra and panties set. Use your favorite porn flicks or erotic stories for inspiration, or flip back to part 7 of this book for classic role-playing ideas.

After setting the scene and getting in character, get going! Act out your fantasy, knowing that the camera is running the whole time. Play to the lens if that excites you; pick up the recorder and move it around to get the best angles. Then let the camera go and lose yourselves in the action, remembering that this is a sex tape—it should be sensual, not silly. Later, settle in for a viewing. Watching yourselves may be nerve-wracking at first, especially if you're focused on how your bodies look. Shut off that voice in your head that's pointing out your cellulite or his love handles, and shift your attention to the act itself. Talk about it: Do you love it when he caresses your thighs or nips at your nipples? Does the way you look up at him during a blow job get him all hot and bothered? Use this as an opportunity to revel in the action, without judging your performance. We recommend deleting the recording afterward—you don't want it showing up on a DVD of family vacation shots—but remember that you can make new "home movies" whenever you like.

Of course, sex tapes aren't always a great idea. Lisa and Harry, for example, will never make a tape—they'd rather not have it end up for sale on the Internet, as has happened to so many other celebs. If you're worried about a sex tape falling into the wrong hands (whether that's a tabloid reporter's or your child's) but still want the thrill, you can act out a sexy scenario but keep the camcorder off. Think of it as a prop for your pretend porn, for your partner's eyes, in real-time only.

FIVE THINGS PORN GETS WRONG

They say art imitates life. Well, not always. Here are our top five gripes with porn.

1. Unrealistic people. Most mainstream porn is filled with young, tanned women with flat stomachs and oversize breasts. The men may not be held to the same standards of so-called perfection, but they usually sport larger-than-average penises. And no one has any hair down there!

2. Constant novelty. We're all for experimenting with acrobatic positions and exciting new venues for sex. But keep in mind that while it might not be the norm in porn, there's a lot to be said for comfort sex.

3. No lube. For the most part, guys just slide right into their wet-and-ready female partners—no assistance required. Yet women often don't immediately lubricate naturally. A bottle of lube can be your best friend, especially during vaginal and anal intercourse.

4. Subpar oral. Don't get us wrong. We like that porn often portrays women on the receiving end of oral sex. At the same time, we're not so impressed with the actors' skills, which sometimes resemble an attempt at tongue fencing rather than a languorous session of oral pleasure. Slow down, guys!

5. Easy orgasms. Research suggests that only about a third of women climax through intercourse alone, but you'd never know it from watching porn. Show us more options for the Big O, please.

FIVE THINGS PORN GETS RIGHT

Porn may not be perfect, but it can still teach us some valuable lessons about sex. Here's what it's doing right.

1. Variety. While you may not want to swing from the chandelier every day, porn can inspire couples to try new positions and act out different role-playing scenarios—and there's nothing wrong with introducing a little exploration into your sex life.

2. Foreplay. We'd like to see more opportunities for women to climax in situations other than intercourse, but porn does portray oral pleasure, manual stimulation, and sex toys, all of which can help take real-life women over the edge.

3. Fantasy. Porn does a great job of giving otherwise shy folks the chance to vicariously live out their wildest dreams. Maybe you and your partner would never actually have a threesome or try anal or experiment with bondage; porn allows you to experience the thrill of such activities without the risk.

4. Visually appealing. Sure, a lot of porn is nothing but bare-bones scenes of sex acts—and there's nothing wrong with that. But some couples, and women in particular, prefer to watch porn that seems less like, well, porn. These days, you can find a wide selection of high-quality films that have good production values, attractive actors, and even actual plots. For a list of suggestions, see "Favorite Flicks" on page 206.

5. Something for everyone. Whether you're into mainstream guy-on-girl action or niche fetish flicks, there's a huge variety of porn available to suit your fancy.

ian says . . . VIVA LA VULVA

Vajazzling. Bikini waxing stencils. Vaginal "rejuvenation" surgery. There are loads of products and procedures out there that exist solely to make a woman's genitals prettier or cleaner or odorless or extra tight. But do you really need to feel self-conscious about yet another part of your body? And what's causing this flare-up of low female genital self-esteem, anyway?

A lot of it is due to cultural pressure—and it starts with porn. In addition to surgically enhanced breasts and bleached blond hair, porn stars are also sporting designer vulvas, leading men and women everywhere to believe that all genitals should look the same. And the beauty and plastic surgery industries don't help. Along with the things listed above, and in addition to labiaplasty and vaginal rejuvenation surgery, some spas are even offering vulva facials, a service that only compounds the idea that women's labia need some extra help.

And many men aren't helping, either. In addition to holding up porn stars as their erotic ideal, some men say they find "imperfect" genitalia ("imperfect" meaning that the inner lips protrude beyond the outer lips) a turnoff, as they believe it indicates a woman has been around the block a time or two. This belief is simply not based in fact and is not true. Still, even male medical professionals are pushing for women to undergo labiaplasty. In fact, a study published in the *Journal of Sexual Medicine* found that male physicians are more likely than female physicians to recommend the surgery. It's no wonder so many women are feeling self-conscious, and seriously considering this intrusive procedure.

Why should women think twice before considering labiaplasty or other procedures such as "labial puffs"? For one thing, labia come in all shapes and sizes. They're not typically symmetrical, and it's incredibly common for the inner labia to protrude beyond the outer labia. So if you think your vulva looks a little bit different . . . of course it does! There are as many styles of vulva as there are women who walk the earth.

Not only that, but because your labia are full of nerve endings, labiaplasty may actually lessen your chances of ever reaching orgasm, and could even make sex painful. Considering that it's sometimes tough enough for a woman to reach orgasm—especially through intercourse alone—it seems silly to lessen those odds even further. And there may even be some benefit to having longer labia minora: They can increase friction during intercourse, which can in turn increase pleasure for both you and your partner.

So the verdict on labiaplasty? Leave your labia alone—they're fine just the way they are. And as for those guys out there who would refer pejoratively to a woman's labia or insist that she wax her vulva until it resembles a plucked chicken, I say leave the boys to their porn and know that there are plenty of men out there who appreciate and savor a woman's natural genital beauty and wouldn't want her vulva any other way. As Napoleon wrote in a love letter to Josephine: "A thousand kisses to your neck, your breasts, and lower down, much lower down, that little black forest I love so well."

coping with

FEMALE
SEXUAL
ISSUES

I t's clear that confidence is crucial for a good love life, but it's tough to feel self-assured when you're coping with a sexual problem. We'll talk about some common male sexual dysfunctions in part 10 of this book, but guys aren't the only ones who can experience obstacles between the sheets. Women have their own share of potential sexual issues, too, including low libido, painful sex, and difficulty reaching orgasm.

These and similar issues are often lumped under the umbrella term "female sexual dysfunction." Sounds official, right? And according to a well-publicized 1999 study in the *Journal of the American Medical Association*, some 43 percent of American women have experienced sexual dysfunction. The problem is that there's no clear definition of female sexual function, or FSD, which makes it hard to determine whether a woman needs "treatment" or whether a particular sexual issue is just another difference between male and female sexuality.

In fact, no one really knows what FSD is. Some people liken it to male sexual dysfunction, but that's just not a valid comparison. It's easy to tell when a man has premature ejaculation or erectile dysfunction, for example. Female sexuality is less obvious. Women just don't always show clear-cut physical signals when they're aroused.

Another reason that FSD is tough to define is because we tend to label men who don't climax during sex as "dysfunctional." Yet more than two-thirds of women don't orgasm from intercourse alone, which suggests that this is normal, not dysfunctional. Even researchers can't agree: In 2000, the *Journal of Urology* offered a few definitions for FSD, including:

- Lack of interest in sexual activity

- "Phobic avoidance" of sexual contact with a partner

- Inability to attain or maintain sexual excitement

- Difficulty attaining orgasm

- Genital pain or pain during intercourse

More than a decade later, though, there's still no consensus on which, if any, of these definitions is accurate. And experts aren't the only ones who are confused: Although studies suggest that the drug flibanserin could be the new "female Viagra," the FDA recently declined to approve its use, saying it failed to completely prove efficacy in treating FSD.

Some critics say we shouldn't be "medicalizing" sex at all and don't need a pill to treat a condition that may not even exist. After all, lots of women often simply aren't in the mood for sex, or are distracted by life's stresses, or just need to start using lubricant. That doesn't mean they're dysfunctional. And other researchers have criticized the "43 percent" statistic in the years since it was published: They point out, for instance, that the women were only followed for two months—suggesting that they could have been experiencing temporary difficulties, not lasting dysfunction—and that the women were never asked whether their sexual issues caused them distress.

Actually, many of these women may be perfectly normal: More recent data from the Kinsey Institute suggest that a woman's emotional health and personal relationship play a bigger role in her sexual satisfaction than her ability to climax. And sex researcher Rosemary Basson, M.D., has proposed a new framework for thinking about female sexual response, which places the importance of emotional intimacy and relationship satisfaction at its center. Dr. Basson's framework contends that female sexual arousal is more complex than a male's and depends more intensely on factors such as relationship satisfaction, self-esteem, and previous sexual experiences. Maybe comparing male and female sexuality isn't quite like comparing apples and oranges—but it might be a bit like comparing oranges and, say, tangerines. They're similar, but they've got some distinct differences.

We believe that the issue of FSD isn't black and white. Sure, FSD isn't as physically obvious as male sexual problems. But that doesn't mean that FSD doesn't have a physiological component, too. Side effects of medications (including some antidepressants, blood pressure drugs, and birth-control pills), shifting levels of hormones, stress and anxiety, obesity, and conditions including diabetes and multiple sclerosis can all lower a woman's desire. So FSD—if it indeed exists—isn't simply perception, just as it's not totally physical. It could be a combination of brain *and* body—although whether a drug can effectively treat FSD remains unseen.

Yet there are undoubtedly issues that can interfere with your sex life. We've already talked about difficulties achieving orgasm in part 6. Three other problems—low sexual desire, trouble with sexual arousal, and painful sex—also commonly affect women. These issues must cause a woman distress to technically be considered "dysfunctions." If you think you may be experiencing one or more of these difficulties, read on. And remember, sexual issues don't have to be a bummer. Just because you're dealing with a problem now doesn't mean that it will last forever, or that it has to put a crimp in your sex life. When you start to view sexual challenges not as roadblocks but as opportunities, you give yourself permission to relax, let go, and even have fun as you tackle them. The tips in this section can help you do just that.

NOT TONIGHT, DEAR: COPING WITH LOW LIBIDO

Just not feeling it lately? Does it seem like your sex drive is stalled out? A lot of women (and men, too) experience dips in their libido over time. There's actually a name for the "condition" of low female sexual desire: hypoactive sexual desire disorder, or HSSD. It's defined as a type of sexual dysfunction in which a woman experiences a persistent or recurrent absence of sexual fantasy, sexual desire, and/or receptivity to sexual activity, which causes personal distress. Although some sources claim that HSDD affects about 40 percent of women, that statistic only means that 40 percent of women have experienced low sexual desire at some point in their lives. (Frankly, we're surprised that number isn't higher!) When you look at those who have ongoing, chronic problems with low sex drive, however, HSDD affects closer to 5 to 15 percent of women.

Many of the reasons for this decreased lack of interest are completely normal, but if they have lasting effects on your libido, you could be diagnosed with HSSD. Research suggests that HSSD (and decreased sex drive in general) can have a wide range of causes: According to a study in the October 2010 issue of the *Journal of Sexual Medicine*, 85 percent of women with HSSD report physical or emotional triggers for the problem, including:

STRESS. Stress may the number-one culprit in low sexual desire for both men and women. Too much of it can sap your libido by affecting hormones, energy, and mood, and by interfering with the quality time that helps a couple stay connected. The relaxation techniques and other stress-busting measures mentioned throughout this book can help you both feel less frazzled.

PHYSICAL HEALTH. A healthy sex drive has both emotional and physical aspects. The physical causes of low desire may include low levels of the sex hormone testosterone due to aging, menopause, or recent childbirth; fatigue; certain medications, such as many antidepressants, drugs used to treat high blood pressure, and birth-control pills (see "A Bitter Pill?" on page 221); conditions that can interfere with your self-esteem, such as incontinence; and other chronic diseases such as heart disease, diabetes, and arthritis. If you suspect that a physical problem may be responsible for your flagging libido, see your doctor.

MENOPAUSE. The hormonal shifts that accompany menopause can affect your desire for sex on many levels. The ovaries stop functioning, causing levels of estrogen, testosterone, and progesterone to decline. Low estrogen levels can cause vaginal dryness and pain during intercourse, while low testosterone levels may trigger changes in sexual desire. Plus, depression and other emotional changes can make you feel less than sexy. We'll talk more about how menopause can affect your sex life in part 12 of this book.

EMOTIONAL ISSUES. Depression, anxiety, relationship conflict and anger, past trauma or abuse, issues with self-esteem or body image, and other emotional woes can all affect your libido. Postpartum depression can also play havoc with your sex drive, as Lisa describes in part 11. Low sexual desire also may occur because of other sexual function complaints, such as trouble with arousal, difficulty achieving orgasm, or painful intercourse, since they can turn sex into a source of stress, not pleasure. In these cases, you might find it helpful to see a therapist, sex counselor, or other health professional, either alone or with your partner.

Just because low libido has an official-sounding name doesn't mean that it requires medical treatment. There are plenty of nondrug options for boosting desire: Make sure you're following healthy lifestyle measures like getting regular exercise, eating a wholesome diet, and managing stress. (For more details on getting sexually fit, see part 4.) Talk to your partner about how you're feeling, and consider counseling either alone or together if you think it may help. Make sex a priority by scheduling couple time—even if you don't have sex, you can still increase your intimacy in other ways, like kissing, cuddling, and touching, which can actually be a real bonus for both of you. If your doctor does recommend pharmaceutical treatment, it may be in the form of supplemental testosterone. It's not for everyone: The FDA hasn't approved testosterone replacement for use in women, and too much of the hormone may cause side effects such as acne, excess body hair, and mood changes. Testosterone may be most effective for women who have had their ovaries removed surgically.

A BITTER PILL?

If you take birth-control pills and have noticed a drop in your libido, you're not imagining things. In fact, oral contraceptives can lower your levels of testosterone, a sex hormone produced by your adrenal glands and ovaries and necessary for desire. Women have only about 10 percent of the testosterone that men do, but it's crucial for a healthy libido and for sexual fantasies. When you take the Pill, your amount of sex hormone-binding globulin (SHBG) can increase by 200 to 400 percent. SHBG binds to testosterone, which means that it isn't available to the rest of your body. As a result, your desire drops, along with your frequency of sexual fantasies and ability to lubricate. Worse, SHBG can remain high in your body, even two years after you stop taking birth-control pills—and your sex drive can take at least as long to recover. And because your level of testosterone naturally begins to decrease as you age, this can become a real problem for women in their thirties and forties. "After about eighteen years, I finally went off the Pill when my second daughter was conceived," Lisa admits. "The difference in my libido was unbelievable! I went from feeling like I'd been living in a convent to wanting sex much more often."

If you think that the Pill (or vaginal rings, which also sap testosterone) seems to be affecting your libido, check with your doctor about suitable alternatives. Some women find that simply changing the type of oral contraceptive they take can help—triphasic pills that contain different amounts of hormones every week may be less problematic, for example.

NOTHING DOING: SEXUAL AROUSAL PROBLEMS

Low sexual desire is very common in women. But what if you have a problem with arousal? You *want* to drive the car, but you're out of fuel and there's no gas station in sight. Persistent arousal difficulties used to be given the rather insulting diagnosis of "frigidity." These days, such problems are labeled female sexual arousal disorder (FSAD), but only if a woman finds them personally distressing. Symptoms may include a lack of psychological excitement, or a lack of vaginal lubrication, genital sensation, and other physical responses after sexual stimulation.

FSAD may be caused by a variety of issues, including a lack of information about your body, sex, or sexual response; poor blood flow caused by high blood pressure or cardiovascular disease; nerve damage from diabetes or pelvic surgery; declining hormones around the time of menopause; certain medications such as antidepressants, antihypertensives, and sedatives; and psychological issues such as a history of sexual abuse, stress, anxiety, depression, addiction, a lack of attraction, or unresolved hostility in a relationship.

As you can see, FSAD and HSSD have many of the same triggers. Perhaps that's because female desire and arousal are closely linked, and both have physical and psychological components. You might not be able to tell the difference easily: Research even suggests that many women have sex before they're actually physically aroused, even though they may think they are. In fact, arousal issues give you a great opportunity to start experimenting with racy activities you might not have previously considered, such as using lubricants and vibrators during sex play, erotica and porn, Kegel exercises, and female arousal gels (such as K-Y INTENSE and Zestra) to help increase blood flow to the genitals. Your doctor may also recommend the EROS clitoral therapy device, a small, FDA-approved vacuum pump that, when placed over the clitoris, provides gentle suction that increases blood flow and arousal.

WHEN SEX IS A PAIN

If you have a vagina, you've probably experienced painful sex at least once. Most women feel pain the first time they have intercourse, for example, although this sensation usually eases with time, practice, and knowledge of their body and their partner. Other women have a recurring problem with discomfort or pain during sex. In fact, nearly one in three women experience pain during sex, according to the recent National Survey of Sexual Health. Sensations of pain can range from dull, to throbbing, to a burning or tenderness of the skin. Some women experience pain during intercourse, others after intercourse. As you might imagine, painful sex can have negative effects on your relationship: You might start avoiding all kinds of intimacy with the fear that it will lead to sex, and both you and your partner can feel hurt and frustrated as a result. It can be difficult to talk about, but sharing your feelings with your partner can prevent confusion and help him understand that you can work together as a team to find a solution.

Pain or discomfort related to sex can have many causes, both temporary and chronic; fortunately, most of them are treatable:

VAGINAL DRYNESS. This is a common culprit in painful sex and is easily remedied with additional lubricant (see part 3 for details) or by spending more time on foreplay to reach maximum arousal before intercourse. If you're not aroused enough, your vagina won't fully expand, which means that your guy could hit your cervix with his penis while he's thrusting, another source of pain. Sex with a partner whose penis is larger than average can also be uncomfortable, particularly if you're not used to it.

INFECTION. If you're sufficiently aroused and are using lube but still feel pain, you could have an infection. Both urinary tract infections and reproductive tract infections can cause pain, and may have no other symptoms.

UNDERLYING HEALTH ISSUES. Some common causes of uncomfortable or painful penetration are underlying health issues that require treatment beyond foreplay and a lubricant. These include endometriosis; a tipped or retroverted uterus; scar tissue from a C-section, hysterectomy, or other pelvic surgery; and interstitial cystitis.

lisa says . . . COMING CLEAN WITH YOUR PARTNER

If you're not feeling up to sex—whether because your desire is practically nonexistent, you have trouble climaxing, or you're coping with one or more of the many other issues that can put a crimp in your sex life—you're not alone. I've already written pretty candidly here about my own struggle with "getting my sexy back" after the birth of my daughters. And if I've learned anything, it's that you just can't suffer in silence.

Fessing up to a sexual issue isn't easy—in fact, it can seem like one of the hardest things to do, even when you love and trust your partner. But the alternative is worse: You're in a slump but your guy is still raring to go, and he may start to wonder if you've stopped being attracted to him. That's why communication is key. I told Harry I had something important to discuss with him—and then I spilled it. I knew I had lost my mojo and not only did I want my husband to know that it wasn't because of him, but I needed his help to get it back.

Harry was surprised, but grateful for my honesty. As difficult as the idea of that conversation had seemed, the reality was a big game changer for us. My confession transformed low sexual desire from "my" problem to "our" challenge—one that Harry was only too happy to help me overcome. And that was the first step in a journey to reclaim our sex life, which, I'm thrilled to report, is hotter than ever. So open up to your partner and start working on your sexual issues as a team. The results are worth it!

HORMONAL CHANGES. Many women experience pain as a result of hormonal changes during menopause and after childbirth, especially if they are breast-feeding.

TIGHTENING UP. If you're nervous, anxious, stressed out, unsure, or inexperienced, your pelvic muscles can tense up, making intercourse painful. When this problem is chronic and prevents penetration altogether, it's called vaginismus.

You can help ease the way by waiting to have sex until you're relaxed and by taking deep breaths during penetration. If the problem persists, see your doctor.

VULVODYNIA. While relatively rare, this chronic condition describes pain that occurs in a variety of scenarios, not just intercourse: when he puts his finger inside you, when you insert a tampon, even when you wear tight pants. Vulvodynia requires diagnosis and treatment by a physician knowledgeable about it.

For the most part, you can prevent discomfort during intercourse by using the tricks in this book to increase your arousal and by using lubricant. If you're still experiencing pain, pay a visit to your health-care provider for a complete physical.

THE TRUTH ABOUT FEMALE VIAGRA

Guys have their "little blue pill"—shouldn't women have a pink version? The pharmaceutical industry sure seems to think so. In the years since the successful 1998 launch of Viagra to treat erectile dysfunction, scientists have scrambled to find a similar medication to boost female sexual desire and arousal. When studies showed that Viagra itself is ineffective in women, researchers turned to other options.

Most recently, the focus has been on flibanserin, a drug aimed at increasing levels of serotonin and other neurotransmitters linked to sexuality. Yes, some women who took it in trials reported a modest increase in sexual satisfaction, but the Food and Drug Administration has not approved the drug, pointing to other studies that show flibanserin failed to increase sexual desire in women significantly enough to warrant the daily use required for this medication.

Part of the problem may be that in general, women's sexual desire and arousal just aren't the same as men's. It may be difficult—and perhaps impossible—to replicate the effects of a male sexual treatment in women. For now, there's no magic bullet to boost your desire—except for maybe a bullet vibrator.

part ten

·

coping with
MALE
SEXUAL
ISSUES

*e*ver wish you had a direct line of communication with your guy's penis? Instead of wondering whether he just wasn't that into you, you would know when his behavior in the sack was really caused by a sexual health issue—and how to help him deal with it. Of course, penises can't talk. (Really, that would be kind of . . . weird.) But guys themselves aren't much better at discussing these topics, either. Let's face it: Even the most emotionally evolved men aren't typically clamoring to share their sexual concerns with the women in their lives. It's not surprising, then, that this lack of communication leaves a lot of women feeling hurt and confused. For all the talk about how "complicated" women's sexuality is, men—and their bodies—are pretty difficult to decipher as well.

That's why a book about sex wouldn't be complete without a section on understanding male sexual issues. With a little knowledge and patience, you can feel confident talking to your guy about potential problems and understand how to work with him to achieve a satisfying—and steamy—sex life. Think of the following chapters as additional tools in your relationship tool kit. Like female sexual problems, male sexual issues don't have to have a negative effect on your sex life. Yes, they can be challenging, but they can also present an excellent opportunity for you and your partner to broaden your bedroom horizons by trying new things together. Even if your partner doesn't currently have a sexual issue, the information here can help you know what to look for if problems arise in the future—and you might just discover some fun new tips to try out now.

TALKING ABOUT MALE SEXUAL PROBLEMS

Sexual concerns aren't just a man's issue—they're a couple's issue. You can't solve your guy's specific problem for him, but your support and understanding can go a long way to helping him deal with it. Of course, addressing sexual problems can be awkward. The best time to talk about sex is when you're *not* having sex—chatting while you're "in the moment" can stop the action right in its tracks. Instead, wait until you're outside the bedroom, in a non-sexual setting. Start by reassuring your guy that you enjoy your sex life and your relationship as a whole. Tell him that you've been doing some reading about his particular issue and that you've learned that there are many different causes and triggers, as well as many different treatment options. Ask him if he'd like to see what you've been reading or discuss it with you. If he's open to it, share the information in this with him.

17

UP FOR ANYTHING? DEALING WITH ERECTILE DISORDERS

Staff. Rod. Throbbing member. If romance novels are any indication, an aroused man means a rock-hard erection. But that's not always the case in real life. Fiction is fiction for a reason, and the truth is that most women have had the disappointing experience of reaching down to cop a feel in the heat of passion, only to grab a penis that's a little too soft for their liking. Or a guy starts out with an erection but loses it when it matters most: during sex. Such problems are quite common: According to the results of the Global Better Sex Survey, published in the April 2008 issue of the *Journal of Sexual Medicine,* 65 percent of men aren't satisfied with the quality of erections (and neither are 63 percent of women).

You might worry that his inability to "get it up" is a sign that he's just not into you. But things are rarely that clear-cut. Erectile disorders typically have very little to do with your attractiveness to a man. Instead, they can have a wide variety of causes, including physical conditions that limit blood flow to the penis or damage the nerves in the area, low testosterone, alcohol consumption, stress, depression, and anxiety.

Of course, it's normal for guys to occasionally have difficulty getting or staying hard—they're not machines, after all. When that happens, we recommend assuring him that it's not a concern and moving on to other activities. If a man has erectile problems in more than 25 percent of his sexual encounters over a period of time, however, he may have erectile dysfunction (ED). Erectile problems can occur throughout a man's life but do appear to increase as he gets older: According to the large Massachusetts Male Aging Study, the incidence of ED in men age seventy and older is triple that found in forty-year-old men. Other research suggests that half of all men between the ages of seventy and seventy-eight have ED, compared to 20 percent of men in their fifties. That's often due to physical problems such as high blood pressure, atherosclerosis, and heart disease, which decrease blood flow to the penis and raise the risk of ED. But ED isn't unusual in younger men, in which case issues like performance anxiety, alcohol consumption, and overuse of pornography (and, consequently, over-masturbation) are more likely to play a role.

THE HARD FACTS ABOUT ED TREATMENT

Your support can go a long way in helping your partner get treated for ED. In a study published in the November 2009 issue of the *Journal of Sexual Medicine,* for example, researchers found that men were more likely to seek help for ED if their female partners were satisfied with the relationship before ED began and had a positive attitude about treatment. Treatment can benefit you, too: A study in the November 2010 issue of the same journal found that women felt that their relationships were more loving and stable and less stressful and that their emotional closeness and communication had improved after their male partners were treated for ED. Here's a look at the most common treatment options for ED:

■ PHOSPHODIESTERASE INHIBITORS. Currently, three oral medications—sildenafil (Viagra), tadalafil (Cialis), and vardenafil (Levitra)—can help treat ED. All three belong to a class of drugs called phosphodiesterase inhibitors and enhance the effects of nitric oxide, a chemical that a man's body produces to relax the muscles in his penis. ED drugs make it easier for a man to get and keep an erection. These medications differ slightly (Viagra and Levitra take effect in about thirty minutes and last four to five hours; Cialis works in about fifteen minutes and can last up to thirty-six hours), but they all have similar side effects, such as headaches, stuffy nose, and blurry vision, and shouldn't be taken by men who have had a recent stroke or heart attack or who take nitroglycerin drugs. Phosphodiesterase inhibitors appear to improve ED in about 65 to 70 percent of men who take them.

- **ALPROSTADIL.** This medication can be injected directly into the shaft of his penis or inserted into the penis in the form of suppositories. Both forms of alprostadil work by increasing blood flow to the penis. Although very effective, they can be painful and result in scar tissue.

- **TESTOSTERONE.** Patches, creams, or injections of testosterone may help men whose ED is caused by low levels of this hormone.

- **PENILE IMPLANTS.** Once the mainstay of ED before the advent of oral-drug treatment, penile implants are surgically inserted into the spongy tissue of the penis, where they remain permanently. Studies show that 70 to 80 percent of men are satisfied with their penile implants, which makes them a useful option for men who can't take ED medications.

- **PENIS PUMPS.** This hollow tube fits over a man's penis and requires either a hand- or battery-powered pump to create a vacuum that draws the blood into the penis, resulting in an erection. The man then applies a constriction device (penis ring) at the base of his penis and removes the tube. Pumps and penis rings can be effective temporarily but may cause pain, bruising, and difficulty ejaculating.

- **COUNSELING.** If his ED has a psychological cause, a sex therapist may help. Look for one who is certified by the American Association of Sexuality Educators, Counselors and Therapists (AASECT). Experts with this certification have had training related to both relationship issues and sexual concerns.

Conventional treatments can help, but there are ways to cope with ED from between the sheets, too. These approaches can actually spice up your sex life, because they let your guy enjoy more oral and manual stimulation (something most men are happy to oblige!) and put the focus on foreplay, which most women crave anyway:

- **GIVE HIM A REST.** When a man is on top during sex, he may put extra stress on the large muscle groups of his thighs and glutes, which sends more blood flow to these areas and takes it away from the pelvis and penis. Get on top and let him lie on his back, or try lying on your sides, either facing each other or spooning, to keep the blood flowing to his erection.

- **USE YOUR MOUTH AND HANDS.** Giving a man oral sex with suction can act similarly to a vacuum pump, especially if you use your hand and add mild pressure at the base of his penis.

- **MIX IT UP.** Oral sex, manual stimulation, vibrators, and other sex toys give you plenty of fun options to choose from that don't rely solely on an erection for pleasure, making ED less of an issue.

18

COMINGS
AND GOINGS:
EJACULATION ISSUES

Like penis size, ejaculation can be a source of pride for men. (Just think about the climactic "money shot" in porn.) Unless they're trying to get pregnant, though, most women don't much care about ejaculation—until it happens too soon or not at all.

To understand how problems can occur, it helps to understand how ejaculation works in the first place. Simply put, ejaculation is the release of seminal fluid from a man's body and a by-product of his orgasm. But ejaculation isn't just about his penis and other reproductive organs. It involves his nervous system, too. Actually, we have two types of nervous systems—sympathetic and parasympathetic—and different parts of his arousal fall within these types. The sympathetic nervous system controls the body's stress-related functions such as the "fight or flight" response, which allowed our caveman ancestors to battle or escape dangerous predators, while the parasympathetic nervous system controls lower blood pressure, a slower heartbeat, and other functions related to relaxation.

The process of ejaculation begins when a guy is sexually aroused. His brain responds by sending signals to his lower spinal cord, and he gets an erection, thanks to his parasympathetic nervous system. As a result, the muscles in his prostate gland, seminal vesicles (both of which produce seminal fluid), and vas deferens (the tube that connects the testicles to the urethra) contract rhythmically, moving semen through those glands and the urethra and, finally, out of his body during ejaculation, which is controlled by the sympathetic nervous system. An orgasm is the sensation of pleasure a man feels during ejaculation.

Orgasms are more straightforward for men than they are for women. While it's easy for a woman to "lose" an orgasm even as she's having it, all guys have a point of what's called "ejaculatory inevitability" during sex when they can't hold back from an orgasm, no matter what. All men also have an "ejaculatory threshold," which is the amount of stimulation they can experience before reaching this point of no return. Yes, orgasmic bliss is more of a sure thing for guys, but it's not always a benefit: It's easy for some men to pass that point of ejaculatory inevitability sooner than they—and their partners—would like. That's called premature ejaculation.

SHORTCOMINGS: DEALING WITH PREMATURE EJACULATION

It's happened to most women at least once: You're enjoying hot and heavy sex with a guy; you're *almost* there; just a little bit longer—and then he climaxes, leaving you feeling less than satisfied. It's frustrating, but the truth is that most men occasionally ejaculate sooner than they (and you) would like. When that happens, try not to take it personally or get upset and move on to other sexual activities instead.

Some men, however, *consistently* ejaculate too soon: Sometimes intercourse only lasts mere seconds, if they make it that far. If this sounds familiar, your guy could have premature ejaculation (PE). According to the International Society for Sexual Medicine, PE is "a male sexual dysfunction characterized by ejaculation that always or nearly always occurs prior to or within about one minute of vaginal penetration; inability to delay ejaculation on all or nearly all vaginal penetrations; and negative personal consequences, such as distress, bother, frustration and/or the avoidance of sexual intimacy." Although more studies are needed, research suggests that this new definition of PE may affect about 30 percent of men at some point in their lives.

Some men have acquired, or situational PE, which means that they develop PE over time. Acquired PE can be caused by psychological or relationship concerns or by physical conditions such as erectile dysfunction and prostate problems. For many guys, though, PE is a chronic problem that they've been dealing with their whole lives. Researchers believe that PE may be partly genetic; it also appears to be influenced by changes in a man's levels of the neurotransmitters dopamine and serotonin, which the nervous system relies on to regulate various bodily functions, including ejaculation. Psychological problems like anxiety and guilt, bad masturbation habits, greater penile sensitivity, and lack of sexual experience may be at least partly responsible for PE.

Sound like your partner? Chronic PE has three main characteristics:

- **QUICK ON THE TRIGGER.** The average guy without PE can only have intercourse for an average of about two to five minutes before ejaculating. For men with PE, though, that's an eternity—most can only last about a minute or less before they climax. Researchers use a system called Intravaginal Ejaculatory Latency Time (IELT) to measure how long a man can have intercourse before he ejaculates. In general, men with PE typically last somewhere between fifteen and sixty seconds, and many guys with PE can't even make it to penetration.

- **NO CONTROL.** The old "think about baseball" trick doesn't work for guys with PE. Their biochemistry—that point of no return—means that they can't control or delay ejaculation and often orgasm at or shortly after penetration, whether they want to or not. In general, men with PE can't last long enough to satisfy a woman during vaginal intercourse.

■ **WIDESPREAD EFFECTS.** Men with PE can experience a range of emotions because of their condition: They may feel angry and frustrated, insecure and anxious about their sex life, embarrassed, worried about their relationship, or a combination of these.

TREATMENTS FOR PE

Even the strongest couples can find themselves dealing with the effects of PE: You might feel confused and unsatisfied, he probably feels guilty and embarrassed, and you're both concerned about your shared sex life. But PE doesn't have to be a deal breaker. Although there's no cure for the condition, you and your guy can manage it with a combination of pharmaceutical measures, behavioral changes, and sexual approaches:

■ **ANTIDEPRESSANTS.** Remember the neurotransmitters serotonin and dopamine? Serotonin increases ejaculatory threshold and delays ejaculation and orgasm while dopamine decreases them. We need the right balance of both neurotransmitters for optimal sexual function, but researchers have found that men with PE have lower levels of the neurotransmitter serotonin. A class of antidepressant drugs called selective serotonin reuptake inhibitors or SSRIs increases levels of serotonin. SSRIs require a prescription, only work as long as a man takes them, and can have side effects such as weight gain, headaches, and nervousness.

One SSRI, called dapoxetine hydrochloride (Priligy), is being tested and marketed specifically as a treatment for PE. Like other SSRIs, dapoxetine appears to increase the ejaculatory threshold and

TOP FIVE MYTHS ABOUT PE

Because of the differences between male and female sexuality, and because most guys tend to clam up about sexual dysfunction, women are left to rely on assumptions or guesswork to figure out what's going on. Are *you* guilty of any of these common misconceptions?

1. He wants you—*bad*. At first, PE can seem flattering. You might misinterpret it as an indication that your guy is so passionate that he can't hold back. But the truth is, PE has little or nothing to do with a man's sex partner. It's about him, not you.

2. He's not interested. On the other hand, you may see the way a man deals with PE—avoidance, for example—as a sign that he's just not that into you. That's usually not true, either. Again, it's not always about you!

3. He's selfish in the sack. If you don't know what's going on, it's easy to view his PE as a "wham, bam, thank you, ma'am" approach. Yet men with PE are usually overly sensitive lovers and worry a lot about their performance.

4. He doesn't know what he's doing. When a man doesn't discuss PE, your only exposure to it may be the way it's portrayed in movies or TV shows—usually as an overly horny adolescent who can't control himself. But men with PE can be very experienced, mature, and tuned in to their partners' needs. They just can't translate that into actions.

5. He's boring. Men with PE tend to develop a plan or "script" for sex, which can help them deal with the condition. If you don't know why he's following this routine, though, you might think that he just doesn't like to experiment in bed.

delay orgasm, but because it's short acting, it only needs to be taken "on demand" an hour or so before sex, similarly to Viagra.

A growing body of evidence suggests that dapoxetine can improve PE. One large study published in the October 29, 2009, issue of the *Journal of Sexual Medicine,* for example, found that men with PE lasted up to three to four times longer than men who took a placebo (dummy pill), increasing their IELT from an average of 1.1 minutes to 3.9 or 4.2 minutes, depending on the dose. Although that may not seem like a lot, it can be a big boost for guys with PE and their partners. Another 2009 study that looked at men with PE in twenty-two countries also showed that dapoxetine significantly increased IELT. Side effects, such as nausea, headache, and sleepiness, appear to be mild. Despite such benefits, dapoxetine isn't yet available in the United States, but new research may help the drug get another chance soon.

■ **EXERCISES.** Sex therapists have long recommended two exercises, known as the stop-start technique and the squeeze technique, to manage PE by controlling a man's sexual arousal. In the stop-start technique, you or your partner stimulate his penis until he's close to climaxing, then stop all stimulation and start again. In the squeeze technique, you place your hand so that your thumb is on one side of your man's penis and your index and middle fingers are on the other side. When he feels like he's ready climax, you squeeze, which supposedly quashes his desire and prevents orgasm. These exercises can be effective, but they need to be repeated regularly, can make sex feel more like work, and many women feel uncomfortable practicing them—so they're not our treatment of choice for PE.

■ **DESENSITIZING PRODUCTS.** Products like gels, sprays, and creams can numb the head of a man's penis, dulling sensation and helping him last longer. Men may also wear one or more condoms, or condoms that are thicker or contain topical numbing creams, to extend intercourse. But desensitization doesn't address the underlying causes of PE, so it's only a short-term fix. Plus, some men or their sexual partners may be allergic to the numbing ingredients in these products.

But there's good news. Another numbing spray, called PSD502 or TEMPE (Topical Eutectic Mixture for Premature Ejaculation), appears more effective at treating PE: A study published on April 23, 2009, in *BJU International* found that men with PE who used TEMPE spray five minutes before intercourse increased their IELT from an average of about fifteen seconds to about three minutes. Other research has shown similar findings and suggests that the spray significantly improves ejaculatory control and sexual satisfaction, with minimal side effects (mainly mild skin irritation). TEMPE spray is currently not available in the United States, although its manufacturer plans to submit it for FDA approval soon.

These treatments aren't the only way to address PE. Just because a man has the condition doesn't mean you can't have a satisfying sex life with him. Lots of sexual activities have nothing to do with when a guy ejaculates. Better yet, when you reframe PE as an opportunity for *more* pleasure, it becomes less of a stumbling block and more of a benefit. Here are some fun ideas to try:

- **OUTERCOURSE.** Simply put, outercourse is everything you do in bed *except* intercourse: talking, touching, kissing, rubbing, oral sex—basically, foreplay. A guy can put the focus on foreplay to get you hot and bothered, then finish off with some intercourse, a routine many women enjoy.

- **ORAL SEX.** This is one of the most effective ways for many women to climax, but your guy has to know what he's doing! Try raising the issue by following the advice in part 3, or surprise him with a book on the subject, such as Ian's *She Comes First*.

■ **MALE MULTIPLE ORGASMS.** Yup, you read that right: *Male* multiple orgasms. Why should women be the only ones to enjoy coming again and again? For this approach, tell your guy that you want to help him experience the pleasures of multiple orgasms. Your goal is to bring him as close to the edge as possible—just ask him to tell you when he's about to go over. When you bring him close to the point of ejaculatory inevitability without going past it, your partner will experience one or two pleasurable orgasmic contractions, which will release some of the sexual tension that has built up in his pelvic region. Make a fun game out of it and don't worry if he climaxes right away at first. You're not only helping extend his pleasure, but over time, you're helping him learn how to extend yours, too, by increasing his staying power.

■ **PERPENDICULAR POSITIONS.** Certain positions take advantage of the fact that women typically require foreplay and stimulation of their vulva—and the clitoris in particular—to have an orgasm, while the top of a man's penis is less sensitive than the underside. In positions like lying side by side, spooning, and standing, your guy can hold his erect penis in his hand so that it's almost at a right angle to your body and then use it to touch and rub your vulva and clitoris. This can be a big turn-on for you, but also helps him stay in control.

DELAYED EJACULATION:
TOO MUCH STAMINA

Who doesn't want a guy who can keep going all night? Sounds like a lovely fantasy, right? Well, in reality, sex with a man who has seemingly never-ending stamina can be exhausting. Although one sexual stereotype of men is that they climax too soon, a growing number of men suffer from the exact opposite problem: If men consistently have trouble achieving orgasm and ejaculating, they may have an issue called delayed ejaculation (DE). Guys with DE may regularly last upward of thirty minutes (compared to the normal time of two to five minutes), may not be able to ejaculate from intercourse, or may not be able to ejaculate at all. Unlike PE, DE isn't genetic. Instead, it can be triggered by a variety of factors, including antidepressants and other medications, alcohol and drugs, stress and anxiety, control issues, and health problems such as diabetes.

One of the major reasons why DE appears to be on the rise, though, is the rapid proliferation of Internet porn. Easy access to porn has made frequent masturbation more common, which can increase the time it takes for men to reach orgasm and ejaculate during real sex. As you learned in part 8, frequent masturbation can also lead some guys to develop an idiosyncratic masturbatory style, which means they become so accustomed to reaching orgasm through the specific way they masturbate that they have trouble climaxing with a partner.

As a result of DE, men may feel anxious about their sexual performance or have low self-esteem, while the women in their lives may take it personally, question their own attractiveness, or feel angry and resentful. Other women aren't even aware that their partner has DE: The number of men who fake orgasm—which is surprisingly easy to do, especially if they're wearing a condom—appears to be rising right along with DE.

TREATMENTS FOR DE

Fortunately, because DE is mainly triggered by factors within your control, it's pretty easy to manage once a man admits he has a problem with it. Here are some things you and your guy can do to counteract the issue:

- **SEE A DOCTOR.** Your partner should get a clean bill of health to make sure that his DE isn't being caused by an illness or a medication that he takes.

- **GET ON THE WAGON.** Just one or two drinks can significantly delay a man's orgasm. See if reducing the amount of alcohol he consumes improves his DE.

- **STRESS LESS.** Moving his focus away from negative emotions, worries, or concerns and toward the physical sensations he is experiencing during sex can help a man climax more easily. Working with a therapist briefly can also help him deal with stress.

- **PASS UP PORN.** Porn gets guys accustomed to high levels of novelty and stimulation, which can be a problem if your partner is used to climaxing from fantasy more than from reality. We're not saying he has to say no to porn for good, but taking a break for several weeks can help him determine if it's triggering his DE. Invite him to join you in trying the sexy alternatives to porn described in part 8, which will help him better link fantasy with reality.

- **TAKE A MASTURBATION BREAK.** Not only can porn overuse lead to DE, but age can also play a role. As men get older, they naturally tend to experience longer refractory periods (the time between erections), as well as an increased latency period (the time it takes to reach ejaculation). While younger men may be able to masturbate *and* have sex within a few hours or a day, over time it becomes difficult to do both.

So if he's masturbating more than he's having sex, it's time to go "hands off" for a while. When he does masturbate, he can try using his nondominant hand. If he's a righty but switches to his left hand, for example, he won't be able to apply the same levels of physical intensity, so he won't be as physically numbed to the sensations of intercourse.

- **BUILD ANTICIPATION.** Guys who suffer from DE often need a spark of novelty to get them over the edge—and you can help with that. Turn your partner on throughout the day with sexy notes, e-mails, texts, or phone calls that build anticipation and share a fantasy at bedtime to get him even more excited.

- **SAVE THE BEST FOR LAST.** Every guy has his favorite position because of the physical sensation, the view, or the fantasy it provides. So save it for last, when it's more likely to take him over the edge.

19

HIS SEX DRIVE: STALLED OR IN OVERDRIVE?

If you've ever been given the brush-off when trying to get a little action from your guy, you're all too aware that men are just as likely as women to use the old "Not tonight, dear; I have a headache" excuse. In fact, an estimated 10 to 20 percent of men report experiencing low sexual desire, compared to 20 to 30 percent of women. Of course, sometimes a headache (or a backache, or a stomachache, or a long day at work) really is the reason for his disinterest. But often, low male libido has more complex causes, including aging, decreased levels of the sex hormone testosterone, conditions such as heart disease and depression, medications such as SSRIs, and stress. In some cases, a man may not really be suffering from a low sex drive but has been depleting his mojo in other ways, such as masturbating frequently.

Although being constantly turned down by your guy in the bedroom can be a big blow to your self-esteem, a man who truly suffers from a low libido is likely grappling with his own emotions and feeling confused, frustrated, or worried about what's causing his low sex drive. Rather than taking it personally, share these tips with him to help get to the root of the problem:

- **SEE A DOCTOR.** Encourage your guy to visit his physician, who can rule out conditions that commonly deplete sex drive, suggest substitutes for SSRIs or other medications that can affect his libido, and test his blood levels of testosterone.

- **BE HEALTHY.** Stress is a major cause of low sexual desire because it lowers hormones and mood and interferes with the quality time that helps a couple stay connected. That's why it's so important to live a balanced life: He should get enough sleep, eat right, exercise, and manage his time smartly. If he can restructure his daily life to feel more manageable, your sex life and your relationship will benefit.

- **COMPROMISE.** Avoid feelings of rejection or pressure by determining a frequency of sex that works for both of you. The tips in part 2 of this book can help couples with mismatched libido types find common ground.

- **CONSIDER TESTOSTERONE.** Chronic stress, a boring routine, feeling unappreciated at work, a lack of physical activity and exercise, and even some cholesterol-lowering medications can decrease his body's production of the sex hormone testosterone. If changing these lifestyle factors doesn't help, your guy may want to ask his doctor for a blood test to see if his testosterone has dropped, an issue that's quite common as men age. Supplemental testosterone is available as a skin patch, gel, and injection but can have a number of side effects, including decreased sperm production and an enlarged prostate, and should never be used without a doctor's supervision.

ARE YOU IN A SEX SLUMP?

Does your guy really have a low sex drive—or is it just the result of a long-term relationship? As you learned in part 2, those heady hormones that can make us feel so frisky at the beginning of a new relationship typically ebb over time, and sexual desire can become less urgent as a result. Compared to the early days of your relationship, you may feel like you just don't have sex as much as you used to, and that's probably true. Yet committed couples still tend to rate their level of sexual satisfaction as very high, probably because they feel more trusting of and comfortable with each other. Plus, long-term coupledom gives you plenty of practice to find out what works well with each other's bodies. Keep this in mind before automatically assuming that one of you is dealing with a low libido, and start sampling the ideas in this book to give your sex life a boost.

WHEN SEX IS A PROBLEM

Dealing with a man who has a low libido can be frustrating, but the opposite issue presents even more of a challenge. If your partner's engine is revving *all* the time, he could have a problem with sex addiction. Although the term itself is controversial, excessive and impulsive sexual behavior and dependency, or "addiction," is a real issue that can have very real effects on a couple's relationship.

Sex addiction wasn't always well known. In fact, in 2001, when Lisa and her husband, Harry, costarred in *Sex, Lies, and Obsession,* a movie about a couple coping with sex addiction, few people were aware of the problem and it was harder to find good resources and information. These days, though, you don't have to look much further than your copy of *US Weekly* to learn all about bad boys and alleged sex addicts such as Tiger Woods, Jesse James, and David Duchovny. And sex addiction isn't just a celebrity problem: More research is needed, but some studies suggest that 5 to 10 percent of Americans—most of them men—may have some sort of sex addiction or dependency.

In general, sex becomes a problem when it starts to control a man and interfere with his life. It often begins slowly, with solo activities like looking at porn and masturbating. Of course, most guys indulge in those activities and it doesn't make them addicts. From there, though, many sex addicts tend to seek out multiple sexual partners, including prostitutes or escorts, continuing to push the envelope in search of the next big thrill. Their drug of choice is that potent neurochemical cocktail of adrenaline, dopamine, and other feel-good substances that the body releases during sex. Like other addicts, their bad behavior becomes a problem when they continue to pursue it, even at the cost of their relationship, health, safety, and job.

If you suspect your partner might be struggling with sex addiction, watch for warning signs like these:

- He masturbates compulsively, often at the expense of your sex life together

- He consistently accesses and uses pornography

- He cheats on you (often multiple times)

- He practices unsafe sex

- He blames you or other people for his problems, especially in sex

- He denies he has a problem and makes excuses for his actions

- His behavior affects his relationships, his work, or his health

- He engages in phone sex or cybersex with people other than you

- He feels like he can't control his behavior and may feel guilt or shame afterward

HELP FOR SEX ADDICTION

Like other addicts, many people who struggle with sex addiction can be reluctant to admit that they have a problem. Access to e-mail, Internet browsing histories, and other technological footprints make it easy to gather evidence if you suspect your guy has a problem—but you still need to talk about it with him. It's very difficult, but try not to feel betrayed: Sex addicts don't deliberately try to hurt their partners, and the problem has nothing to do with their existing relationship. Instead, discuss these treatment options with him:

- THERAPY. Solo or couples therapists who specialize in treating sex addiction can help both you and your partner learn healthier ways to deal with the issue.

- SUPPORT GROUPS. Group therapy or twelve-step programs like Sex Addicts Anonymous and Sexual Compulsives Anonymous allow men and women to offer and receive support from fellow sex addicts.

- MEDICATIONS. In some cases, medications used to treat obsessive-compulsive disorder may help decrease the compulsive aspects of sex addiction. Drugs that lower libido, such as SSRI antidepressants, are also sometimes used to treat sex addiction.

20

THE SIZE
AND SHAPE
OF THINGS

as the old adage goes, it's not the size of the boat but the motion of the ocean, right? Most women understand that every penis is different and don't get hung up on size, unless a guy's member is unusually small or large. In fact, a research review published in the June 2007 issue of the journal *BJU International* suggests that penis size matters more to *men* than to women: When the researchers looked at more than fifty studies spanning the course of sixty years, they found that 85 percent of women were satisfied with their partner's penis size—yet only 55 percent of men felt good about their penises.

That's a shame, since most men fall into the "average" range, which is determined by penis length (the measurement from the base of a man's penis to the tip) and girth (the distance around a penis, or circumference). Studies suggest that the average erect penis ranges in length between 5.5 and 6.2 inches and between 4.7 and 5.1 inches in girth. Now consider the fact that the average vagina is only about four inches deep during maximal arousal, and you can see why most penises don't pose a problem in terms of your pleasure.

But what if your guy is significantly smaller—or larger—than average? Try these tips.

IF HE HAS A SMALL PENIS

First, remember a simple fact about female anatomy: For most women, the clitoris is more important than the vagina in orgasmic ability, so deep penetration isn't usually necessary. That means that certain types of sex play and positions can be a real benefit for men with smaller penises and their partners:

- **INDULGE IN THE FIRST COURSE.** About 70 percent of women don't climax from intercourse alone, so men need to become skilled in other ways of stimulating their partners, including kissing, touching, sharing fantasies, and stimulating the clitoris manually, orally, or with a vibrator. Another benefit: The opening of the vagina tightens as a woman becomes aroused, making a shorter or thinner erection less of a problem.

- **WORK IT OUT.** Add friction and boost arousal for both of you by using your pelvic floor muscles to squeeze around his penis during intercourse. Make the same movements you would during Kegel exercises (see part 6 of this book for details).

- **TAKE THE LEAD.** Try positions that don't require deep penetration but allow you to grind against his pelvis rather than relying on deep penetration—like "woman on top" and "reverse cowgirl."

- **GO AROUND IN CIRCLES.** When your guy thrusts, he can use more of a circular motion from front to back so that the sides of his erection stretch the opening and the walls of the vagina, which gives you the sensation of experiencing a wider penis. Missionary position is best for this.

IF HE HAS A LARGE PENIS

Bigger isn't always better: A larger-than-average penis can be uncomfortable for some women during vaginal, oral, and anal sex. Here's how to make the experience more pleasurable.

1. **TAKE YOUR TIME.** Although the opening of the vagina tightens as you become aroused, the canal itself expands and lubricates, easing the way for intercourse. Yet many women jump into intercourse before their bodies are ready. The foreplay suggestions for smaller penises apply here, too.

2. **USE LUBE.** Lubricant is absolutely required for couples dealing with a large penis. Experiment with different brands to see what works best for you.

3. **CONTROL THE ACTION.** In general, we recommend positions that let you better control the angle and amount of thrusting and penetration, like "woman on top." You may want to skip those that involve deep penetration, such as rear entry.

quick study: THE MEASURE OF A MAN

We've all heard the old myth: You can tell a guy's penis size simply by looking at his hands, feet, or nose. Believe it or not, researchers have delved into that claim. So where does science stand on the matter? One 1988 study did find a weak relationship between penis size, foot length, and body height, but a 2002 study found no correlation between penis size and shoe size. More recently, a 2011 study concluded that a lower ratio between the length of a man's index finger and the length of his ring finger was associated with a longer penis, but more research is needed to say for sure. If there is a link, scientists suspect it's because the same genes that control the development of the penis also control limb development. For now, the best way to know a guy's penis size is still to take a look.

ian says . . . IS YOUR SEX LIFE IN A RECESSION?

When it comes to a man's sex life, economic woes may be its biggest enemy. The economic turbulence of the past few years has caused couples to cut back on things such as date nights, baby-sitters, gifts to each other, short trips, and of course longer vacations.

Compounding this deprivation, couples are more anxious and stressed than ever about personal finances. In fact, arguments over money remain one of the leading causes of marital strife. So while it may seem counterintuitive to add to your expenses, I strongly suggest that you find a way to put relationship satisfaction at the top of your priority list.

Sure, date night may not seem like a necessity, but like trickle-down economics, a strong relationship fosters personal and professional success. According to anthropologist Helen Fisher, people with healthy sex lives may even do better at work. And a healthy sex life requires a strong underlying relationship to support it.

Financial stress is also a major cause of low libido and sexual dysfunction, especially in men. Desire and sexual confidence stem from self-esteem, which men tend to derive from their jobs and status as providers.

My male clients tend to suffer from sexual issues that are more chronic than "situational," meaning that the person generally has a long history with the problem and that it has a basis in underlying biological, psychological, or relationship issues. But with the volatile state of the economy, many men are reporting sexual issues—such as premature ejaculation, erectile disorder, delayed ejaculation, and low desire—for the first time, or are finding that an occasional issue is suddenly becoming an ongoing problem.

Almost all of these men point to their anxiety over work (or lack thereof), mounting debt, or arguments over money as a main source of their bedroom difficulties. Some of these men begin taking antianxiety medications (which can have their own sexual side effects), but more often they just feel anxious, distracted, depressed, and/or have generally lost their mojo. Sexual dysfunctions are a bit like bedbugs: Once they appear, they're awfully hard to get rid of. Worrying about an issue often becomes a self-fulfilling prophecy.

A recent study in the *Archives of Sexual Behavior* even found that sexual performance anxiety plays a role in male infidelity. According to the study's coauthor, Robin Milhausen, a professor and sexuality researcher at the University of Guelph, "People might seek out high-risk situations to help them become aroused, or they might choose to have sex with a partner outside of their regular relationship because they feel they have an 'out' if the encounter doesn't go well—they don't have to see them again."

Although you might think that a guy who suffers from a sexual issue would be less likely to cheat, that's often not the case. I've seen this dynamic play out many times, especially when a guy blames his partner for the issue or his feeling about the issue is enmeshed with his relationship.

This same study also suggests that women are more likely to cheat because of relationship issues. When a guy is tuned out, turned off, cranky, and critical—as men often are over money issues—a woman is more likely to develop her own doubts about the relationship.

I hope that money won't mess with your relationship. But in my experience, financial issues are about more than just dollars and cents. Money encompasses emotions and family history, and just going through a credit card bill can lead to accusations, generalizations, outbursts, lies, and ultimatums.

People should take a tip from our government, which often takes emergency action to create liquidity and protect the economy. Call the baby-sitter and go on a date night; take that weekend getaway—it's worth it. A recession doesn't have to mean a downward spiral in your love life, and if you invest in your relationship, the return is virtually guaranteed.

part eleven

·

SEX
and
PARENTHOOD

the kids are all right—but what about your sex life? There's no doubt about it: When you have a baby, sex goes from being something that used to be spontaneous to something that goes on an awfully long to-do list. It should be no surprise that studies show that 90 percent of new parents experience a significant decline in relationship satisfaction, and that many couples end up divorced within five years of having a baby. Even if you stay together, you're often so busy raising your kids that between car pools and science projects and play dates and—well, you get the picture!—sex goes out the window.

Of course, we're not suggesting that you ignore your children. Every parent wants his or her child to thrive and be happy. We try to do our best to give our kids everything: time, attention, love. But the fact is that nothing makes children happier than to know that their parents are happy, too. The latest, greatest toy or the richest college fund means nothing to a child compared to seeing his parents hug, kiss, and hold hands. Those little acts can provide a kid with a sense of safety and security that money just can't buy. So don't assume that being a parent means that you have to give up your own happiness. Instead, we want you to get *selfish* about what matters to you as a couple. And that includes a healthy sex life.

From trying to conceive and being pregnant, to having a baby and raising kids, children can dramatically change the face of your relationship. But don't assume that parenthood means celibacy. With an open mind, a little creativity, and your commitment to each other, you and your partner can maintain a smokin' sex life that's different—but maybe even better—than what you had before. Some of the advice in this section also comes from Hilda Hutcherson, M.D., the author of *The Good in Bed Guide to Sex and the Baby Years.*

POP QUIZ

According to OnePoll research, the average couple trying to conceive will have sex how many times before being successful?

(A) Once   **(B)** 10 times   **(C)** 25 times   **(D)** 104 times

Correct Answer: (D) 104 times. Trying to conceive can be incredibly "trying." It's important to communicate and remember that conception sex doesn't have to be goal oriented. You can still enjoy the fun of it.

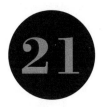

CONCEPTION SEX:
THE BEST-LAID PLANS

For many couples, there is no more exciting time than when they try to conceive a baby. With this goal in mind, sex may at first seem more meaningful and you and your partner may never feel closer. In the beginning, conception sex can also be a time of more freedom: You've given each other permission to have sex whenever you want it, and birth control worries are a thing of the past.

But trying to conceive can also be quite, well, trying. Whether you get pregnant right away, struggle with infertility, or fall somewhere in the middle, sex with the goal of pregnancy isn't always simple. Sure, you can have sex all the time—but that can get a little exhausting, especially for the man, who may start to feel like you only want him for his sperm. You have to schedule intercourse around ovulation, so the sense of spontaneity that can make sex so fun all but disappears. And when you're "doing it" more often, sex can start to seem awfully routine—downright dull, in fact. Add in the potential for both male and female sexual dysfunctions (the risk of which can rise under pressure), and you can see why conception sex can be rife with stressful situations.

Fortunately, you can tackle all of these issues together. According to one recent survey from OnePoll, the average couple has sex 104 times before getting pregnant. So why not make those 104 times feel less like work and more like play?

SEX ON DEMAND. At first, it's a dream come true for many men: a woman who wants sex, wants a lot of it, and wants it *now*. But over time, this "wham, bam, thank you, sir" mentality can wear thin. In fact, one recent survey found that 11 percent of guys complained about sex on demand and admitted to feeling "completely used" during the process. And women can get resentful when men don't do what they want.

One way to deal with the pressure to procreate is to focus on romance, both in and out of bed. Send each other flirty e-mails during the day—not just during ovulation—alluding to all the sexy things you'll do later that night. Help each other out around the house. Hold hands and cuddle. There's no getting around the fact that conception sex will always be about conception, but you can try to make the process more loving. You can also spice up sex on demand with some role-playing by engaging in some mild bondage (try the scenarios in part 7 of this book).

FAKING SPONTANEITY. When you're trying to conceive, your sexual encounters can be dictated in large part by biology. Now your sex life is tied to ovulation, and your appointment book is filled with "dates" for sex. Sex can start to feel like a business transaction.

Maybe you can't control all of the days you have sex, but you *can* mix up what you do: Change the time of day and location of your rendezvous. Try a little role-playing with new names, looks, and personalities for the night. However you spice things up, don't limit yourselves to certain days: Enjoy sex whenever—and wherever—you want it, not just when you're most fertile.

THE SAME OLD, SAME OLD. When you're trying to conceive, sex can start to seem like one more boring task on your to-do list. You might as well be washing the dishes or cleaning the bathroom!

But trying to conceive doesn't have to be a snore or feel like work. Move the focus from conception to the pleasurable sensations that accompany sex.

Enjoy the journey, not just the destination. Buy a new sex toy, wear some sexy lingerie, and touch and kiss each other in less-expected places, like the eyelids, wrists, and ankles.

MALE MALFUNCTIONS. Trying to conceive can pose special challenges for guys. The pressure to perform on demand may eventually rear its head in the form of low sexual desire, erectile dysfunction, premature ejaculation, or delayed ejaculation. Be aware of how conception sex can trigger or worsen these issues, and consult a physician or sex therapist if they don't resolve. For specific advice on these issues, see part 10 of this book.

FEMALE TROUBLES. You might feel excited about the prospect of pregnancy, but that doesn't mean you're immune to various sexual obstacles, too. Sex on demand means that you may be having intercourse before you're truly turned on, so you may experience decreased lubrication and difficulty climaxing as a result. Make sure to focus on foreplay and arousal just as much as usual. And don't forget your orgasm: While you're probably more concerned about his climax (you want that sperm, after all), yours may be just as important. Your orgasm may even help increase your chances of getting pregnant: Some experts believe that the cervical contractions that can accompany climax can pull sperm up the vagina and closer to the egg. While there's little scientific study to prove this theory, having an orgasm might help, and certainly can't hurt, conception. To get there more easily, try to relax, shift the focus away from conception, and stimulate your clitoris, either manually or with positions like "woman on top."

22

AVOIDING A PREGNANT (SEX) PAUSE

Once you become pregnant, your sex life changes—for better or for worse. Now, maybe sex is all you can think about, or it's the last thing on your mind. For many couples, a positive pregnancy test can suddenly shift the focus from conception to the baby itself: Having sex takes a backseat to registering for car seats, as well as having ultrasounds, debating names, and painting nurseries. Other parents-to-be worry that intercourse will hurt the developing baby, so they abstain completely.

The truth is that for most couples, intercourse and other sexual activities are safe throughout pregnancy. Unless your physician, nurse, or midwife has recommended that you abstain from intercourse and/or orgasm, a healthy and satisfying sex life can be beneficial during pregnancy because it keeps you and your partner connected. If you think "pregnancy" and "hot sex" just don't mix, let us help you reconsider.

WHEN *HE'S* NOT IN THE MOOD

It's easy to forget how pregnancy can affect guys, too. Lots of men still find their pregnant partners physically attractive—some even more so. Others simply feel closer to their partner and express that through sex. Yet for every expectant dad who can't get enough, there are others whose desire decreases. Don't worry that it's all about you. There are plenty of other concerns at play, including:

- He's worried he'll hurt the baby (this is virtually impossible).

- He's stressed about money.

- He doesn't want to pressure you.

- He's jealous of the attention you're getting.

- He's scared of change.

Situations like these are why communication is crucial, especially during pregnancy. Share your feelings with your partner and encourage him to talk about his as well. Being able to talk about sex isn't just important now, but for the rest of your lives together, too.

HOW YOUR BODY CHANGES

Pregnancy involves much more than the classic changes of larger breasts, wider hips, stretch marks, and morning sickness. Everyone is different, but pregnancy typically affects sexuality in the following ways:

LIBIDO. In general libido tends to decrease during the first trimester, when pregnancy symptoms can prevent you from feeling sexy. Your sex drive can increase once these symptoms disappear, but may decrease again in the final months of pregnancy. Keep your partner aware of these changes so he doesn't feel confused or rejected.

LUBRICATION. Shifting hormone levels mean you may not lubricate as easily as in the past. Lubrication can increase during the second trimester, though, which may increase your desire for sex.

ORGASMS. The hormonal changes of pregnancy increase blood flow and sensitivity in your genitals, so your orgasms may be even more intense and pleasurable.

SEX WHEN YOU'RE PREGNANT

When it comes to pregnancy sex, the positions you choose can make a big difference in your comfort and pleasure. In general, any position that puts pressure on your back or stomach can be problematic because your baby bump may get in the way. Try these positions instead:

1. **WOMAN ON TOP.** Best for the first and second trimesters, this position can take the pressure off your back and belly and allows you to control the depth and speed of thrusting.

2. **SITTING.** This intimate position allows you to gaze into each other's eyes. It's best during the first and second trimester.

3. **SIDE BY SIDE (FACING).** This intimate position takes the weight off your belly and is best for the first trimester and early second trimester.

4. **SPOONING.** Perfect for the last trimester, this position takes the pressure off your belly and prevents deep penetration, which may be uncomfortable later in pregnancy.

5. **HANDS AND KNEES.** This position can result in deeper penetration, so it's best reserved for the first and second trimesters.

OTHER OPTIONS

You (or your partner) just might not feel comfortable having intercourse when you're expecting. But that shouldn't mean that you avoid *all* forms of intimacy. Sample some of these classics to keep the fires burning:

ORAL SEX. Oral pleasure is totally fine when you're pregnant. As with cunnilingus anytime, just be sure that your partner doesn't blow into your vagina, which can cause an air embolism, which can be life threatening for you and your baby.

TOUCHING. You can indulge in erotic massages, manual stimulation, and mutual masturbation, but remember to add a water-based lubricant. Your breasts may feel particularly sensitive during the first trimester—some women enjoy this, while others find it painful. Tell your partner what you like.

VIBRATORS. Used wisely, vibrators are safe during pregnancy. Choose a battery-powered clitoral massager, use plenty of lube, and don't place a vibe inside your vagina after the second trimester.

lisa says . . . FEELING SEXY WHEN YOU'RE PREGNANT

The way we feel during pregnancy is so individual: Some women may feel sick, uncomfortable, and ungainly. Others have never felt more beautiful. Fortunately for me (and Harry), I was one of the latter. I don't know why. Maybe it was because I knew my body was doing what it was meant to do, or because I was carrying the child my husband and I had conceived together. Whatever the reason, I felt radiant, strong, and, sensual. I wanted to show other women that it's okay—more than okay, actually—to feel sexy when you've got a baby bump. And I wanted men to see that pregnant women can still be gorgeous.

I realize, of course, that not every woman feels good about herself when she's expecting. The side effects and hormonal shifts of pregnancy can make you feel less than hot, even if your man thinks you're smokin'. And those emotions can change from day to day as you progress through the trimesters. I think that the best way to feel sexier is to start getting in touch with your body and treating it right. Take a prenatal yoga class, get a massage, indulge in a mani/pedi, or treat yourself to some of the sexy maternity lingerie available these days. Even a simple candlelit bath spent gently soaping up your belly can make you feel more sensual. And if you and your guy want to stage a session of erotic photography in your own bedroom, go for it! You'll have your own secret keepsakes of this special time.

23

BRAVE NEW WORLD: SEX AFTER KIDS

It's been said that parenthood is the toughest job you'll ever love, and we have to agree. And no matter how much you do love it, having kids will change your relationship in ways you never anticipated, and that includes your sex life. Like it or not, you just won't have the sexual relationship you had before you had a baby: According to a recent survey by the online magazine *Baby Talk,* just 24 percent of parents say they're satisfied with their postbaby sex lives, compared to 66 percent who were happy before they had children. Oof. It's enough to make you never want to procreate.

But there's good news, too: Your sex life can be even better than it was before. Sure, it's going to take some ingenuity and dedication, but it's absolutely possible for both new and longtime parents to enjoy alone time, intimacy—and, yes, hot sex. Trust us: We've both been there. (Lisa and Harry have two daughters, and Ian his wife, Lisa, have two sons.) We totally understand that from those first late-night feedings to the day your kids leave the nest, maintaining a healthy sex life can be incredibly challenging. But we also want you to know that it's not impossible. In fact, over time, you two can grow even closer than ever.

OH, BABY!

In the first weeks (and, sometimes, months) after childbirth, sex is probably the furthest thing from your mind. We don't need to remind you of the obvious: You just had a baby! Chances are, your little one's coos, cries, and—let's face it—screams won't let you forget your new addition anytime soon. Attending to your child's needs takes precedence over your own urges, and that's the way it should be in the beginning.

Eventually, though, even the most frazzled parents need to enjoy intimacy again. Once we have kids, it's way too easy to start thinking of ourselves as just "Mom" and "Dad" and to lose sight of the relationship that we used to enjoy with our partner. We can't stress this enough: You've got to make the effort to build a foundation for intimacy now so you can continue to enjoy a healthy sex life for the rest of your life together.

Of course, it isn't always so easy to plunge back into sex, even if you've gotten the okay from your doctor. Your partner may not be in the mood, either, but women have a particularly difficult time getting back into the sexual swing of things. Several obstacles may be standing in your way:

HORMONAL SHIFTS. The same hormones that spiked when you were pregnant can sink after you give birth, and your libido can suffer as a result. Breastfeeding is great for baby but can send your sex drive even lower, because it triggers your body to release prolactin, a hormone associated with decreased sexual desire.

EXHAUSTION. Good sex requires energy, something that's in short supply when you're caring for a newborn. We can't blame you for choosing sleep over sex. Nap when your baby naps. In time, he or she will develop a regular sleep schedule—and so will you.

BODY IMAGE. Even if you get back to your prepregnancy weight, much of your body—belly, hips, breasts—has changed forever. Keep in mind, though, that

COPING WITH POSTPARTUM DEPRESSION

For many women, a lower libido is the least of their postpregnancy concerns. Quick drops in hormone levels can make you feel weepy and anxious after giving birth. Fortunately, these feelings typically resolve within a few weeks of giving birth. If they last longer, you may have postpartum depression (PPD), a true libido killer. PPD affects about 20 percent of new mothers and can occur any time in the year or so after they give birth. Watch for signs like sadness, lack of energy, trouble concentrating, anxiety, and feelings of guilt and worthlessness. "I've personally struggled with PPD, especially after the birth of my first daughter," says Lisa. "I was thrilled to be a mom, but I also felt sad, confused, and like I didn't know who I was anymore. I suffered in silence for more than a year until I started to feel better, but no one should wait that long to get help." Talk to your mother, your girlfriends, your doctor, and your partner. Ask for help: There are plenty of options available to address PPD, including counseling, support groups, and medicines.

your *vagina* doesn't change: Childbirth won't stretch it out permanently. You may be able to speed its return to its previous size by practicing Kegel exercises (see page 149 for details). Remember, confidence goes a long way in helping you exude sex appeal, so fake that self-esteem until you cultivate it for real.

SELF-IMAGE. In addition to your body, your view of yourself may change as well. You may start seeing yourself only as "Mommy" and not as a sexual being. Be aware of this threat and carve out time for yourself and your partner to avoid losing your sense of self.

TRAUMA. This one's for the guys. Yes, we know what women are going to say: "But *I'm* the one who endured childbirth!" But the event can be fraught with stress for some men who view the process. These men see things—vaginal delivery or C-section—that they wish they hadn't and regret not just staying at the head of the bed holding your hand. Now they may see a body part they once associated with pleasure in a whole new, unsexy light. If you had a C-section, the scar may remind him of watching doctors slice open your abdomen. In either case, it's clear that, for some men, childbirth is a libido killer. Our advice: Just get back in the saddle, guys. Even if you have to go through the motions the first few times around, eventually your arousal hormones will take over and you'll get over your fears.

EASING BACK INTO INTIMACY

Your libido will eventually return, but sex after childbirth can still be nerve-wracking.

When you're ready to try, follow the advice here to help make intercourse more comfortable and pleasurable. Here's what you need for your postpregnancy sexual tool kit:

- PATIENCE. How you physically feel after having a baby is very individual. Some women find that the tenderness caused by vaginal childbirth, episiotomy, or C-section incisions eases quickly, while others require a longer healing period. Even when you get the okay from your doctor, remember to take it slowly. Build arousal by kissing, cuddling, and sharing fantasies before jumping into intercourse.

- LUBRICANT. Decreased levels of estrogen after pregnancy can cause vaginal dryness, as can breastfeeding. Moisturize delicate vaginal tissues by following the advice for lube in part 5 of this book.

- STRENGTH. Pregnancy and childbirth can weaken your pelvic floor muscles. You'll want to strengthen them again, though, because those muscles can make orgasms more intense and increase pleasure for you and your partner. Follow the steps for Kegel exercises on page 149.

Now that you've got the right tools at hand, use them as you begin to reclaim sexual intimacy with your partner:

ENGAGE IN CHOREPLAY. Remember back in part 2, where you learned the value of a bottle of Windex wielded by an enthusiastic partner? Research shows that women need to be able to relax and let go to be able to thoroughly enjoy sex, and "choreplay"—when your guy pitches in around the house—can go a long way in helping you de-stress. Remind him that when he takes some of the tasks off your ever-growing to-do list, sex will make its way closer to the top.

TRY DIFFERENT POSITIONS. Woman on top is a good choice for new moms who are nervous about returning to intercourse because it allows them to control the speed and depth of penetration. Or try side by side or spooning, which takes the pressure off your C-section incision.

BREATHE DEEP. The deep breathing you learned during childbirth classes doesn't just benefit labor. It can also help you relax and focus on pleasure, and may even make your orgasms more intense.

EMBRACE THE QUICKIE. They make baby monitors for a reason. Take advantage of your baby's naptime to get busy in your bedroom, bathroom, kitchen . . . Use the tips in part 5 of this book to build arousal all day so that the payoff is extra hot.

BE INTIMATE. Sex doesn't have to be all or nothing. Even if you're not ready to go all the way, you've got plenty of sensual alternatives to intercourse: Kissing, cuddling, spooning, massaging each other, and enjoying oral pleasure can all help you feel close sexually. Set your boundaries in advance, so you and your partner can relax without worrying about what may or may not lead to intercourse.

DEALING WITH INTERRUPTIONS

The odds are that when you finally do get some much-needed couple time, you're going to be interrupted by your baby. Is she hungry? Does he need a diaper change? Is your child just crying for the heck of it? Whatever the reason, most women have trouble continuing to make love when a little one needs their attention. There's nothing wrong with checking on your baby, but if crying is an ongoing issue, you're going to need to make some adjustments if you want to have sex again anytime soon:

- Determine when your baby sleeps the most. If he tends to be up all night, for example, try having sex in the morning when he's more likely to snooze.

- Time things so that you have sex early into your baby's nap- or bedtime, when she's less likely to interrupt you.

- Give your baby time. You don't need to run to his side every time he cries, a lesson you've probably already learned if you have more than one child.

- Set the mood with soft music that turns you both on and neutralizes normal but distracting baby noises like burping and cooing.

- Forge ahead. If you must get up to tend to your child, make an effort to get back to the sexy scenario at hand once she falls back to sleep. If your partner is waiting for you, send him a naughty text message to tide him over.

- Take turns. Let your partner take care of your baby and relax while you wait for him—taking a hot bath or even reading some erotica can keep you feeling both de-stressed and sensual.

INDULGE IN "ME" TIME. Does anyone feel sexy when she's got spit-up on her shirt and just changed a dirty diaper? We didn't think so. That's why we urge you to get out of the house for a little alone time. Swap child-care duties with your partner or get a sitter, even if it's just for an hour or two. Then treat yourself to a walk outdoors, a trip to the gym, a mani/pedi, a haircut, a massage, or a shopping trip (for you, not your baby). Taking the time and space to reclaim your sense of self can also help you get back in touch with your sensual side.

JUST DO IT. Don't get us wrong. We're not suggesting that you have charity sex just because your partner is in the mood. Give in once in a while, though, and natural arousal will eventually start to follow. Sex begets sex—the more you have it, the more you *want* to have it.

24

STAYING THE COURSE

Our own kids are old enough now that we don't have to worry as much about sneaking in some naptime nooky with our respective spouses. But that doesn't mean that our sex lives have been free of obstacles. Parenthood has its own set of challenges that, if not addressed, can play serious havoc with a relationship. From feeling bored with sex or preoccupied with your work, to looking outside your relationship and indulging in porn, "harmless" flirting, or even infidelity, long-term commitment isn't always easy. Now add in the responsibility of kids—for the next eighteen years, at least—and you've got a potent recipe for some serious sexual problems.

But being a parent and having a healthy sex life don't have to be mutually exclusive. Sure, your role-playing scenarios have likely changed from naughty nurse and dirty doctor to frazzled mommy and daddy. Sex is probably languishing somewhere near the bottom of your to-do list, if it's even on there at all. You're just too . . . busy to get busy. It doesn't have to be that way. It may seem as if you have no time or energy for sex, but it *is* possible to fit in intimacy. Here's how.

MAKE A DATE. It's not exactly spontaneous, but scheduled sex is better than no sex, right? So plan a date night, put it on your calendar, and stick to it. Rather than over-the-top, expensive outings, choose low-key activities that allow you to focus on each other, such as a casual dinner, a movie night at home after your kids are asleep, or a "date day" spent together after you hire a sitter. Reminisce about the early days of your romance. Snuggle as you chat about light topics (absolutely no "kid" talk allowed). Reconnecting like this may naturally lead to sex, or you can raise the stakes with a fun, flirty game (see "Date Night Is in the Cards" on this page).

PUT DOWN THE IPAD. Or the smartphone, laptop, TV remote . . . Everyone needs to unwind at the end of the day, but why relax with Jon Stewart or Angry Birds when you can do it with your partner? Prioritize sex so that you get intimate as soon as the kids are in bed, and *then* load the dishwasher, watch *The Daily Show*, or fall asleep.

Instead of fiddling with your phone in your partner's presence, use that technology during the day to build sexy anticipation. Start with a text that simply says, "I'm thinking of you" or "I wish you were home already." Then amp it up a bit by hinting about a sexy evening together or "sexting" him a nude picture of you. Keep it going throughout the day. By the time you're both home, you'll be ready to fiddle with each other.

try this: DATE NIGHT IS IN THE CARDS

Want an activity for date night? Get yourself a deck of cards and a pack of index cards and settle in for a sexy game of strip poker. Jot down your most sensitive body parts (back of knees, earlobes, breasts, etc.) on half the index cards while your partner does the same with his share. On your other half, each of you should write your favorite types of touch, like a kiss, a tickle, or a caress. Next, place all the index cards in the center of the table, split into two piles: body parts and types of touch. Then play a classic game of poker with the deck of playing cards. If you win, you can choose one index card from the body part pile and one card from the touch pile. Present them to your partner—and ask him to pay up!

FIND THE TIME. Years of parenthood have taught us that you've got to grab time for sex when you can find it. So seize the moment by setting your alarm an hour earlier than usual, taking a "lunch" break together, or sharing a shower together. Fit in a little foreplay in less-expected places such as a dark movie theater, your car, or a public restroom (locked, of course). While you may not go all the way, you'll raise the temperature for sex later on at home.

AVOIDING THE DREADED SEX RUT

We've all been there: You're driving along, enjoying a smooth ride, when suddenly you hit a pothole. Whether you can get out of that rut—or maneuver around it altogether—depends a lot on your vehicle and your driving skills. And if you're not careful, you can seriously damage your car.

lisa says . . . QUICK GETAWAY

From the time our first daughter was about six months old, Harry and I knew that we were going to need to get away for some occasional "couple time" if we wanted to keep our sex life sexy. While you can certainly fit in some quickies at home, there's something about getting out of the house—and away from all of the stress of daily life—that helps you reconnect sexually. Isn't that why vacation sex is so great? You remove yourself from your usual routine, so it's much easier to relax and let go. That's why we try to schedule an overnight date every few months and head out to a hotel. Not only do we get that time together, but it's a great opportunity to dabble in role-playing or other fun, sexy scenarios that aren't always possible at home. If you choose this path, try to start early: Our girls have seen us leave the house for "special time to talk" since they were babies. They get to have a sleepover with their nanny or grandparents and friends and Harry and I get our own, very private party!

Automotive analogies aside, life is filled with metaphorical roadblocks, and your sex life is no exception. Most couples—forty-one million Americans, according to some estimates—fall into a sex rut from time to time, and parenthood doesn't make avoiding them any easier. Over time, a simple rut can become an enormous sinkhole. In fact, one recent poll by NBC *Today* found that 30 percent of all people have gone a few months without sex—and 22 percent have gone a whole year. It makes sense when you think about it: The less you have sex, the less you want it. When you're in a dry spell, your levels of the sex hormone testosterone drop, taking your libido with them.

Fortunately, *more* sex can boost your sex drive. Like exercise, it can be hard to find the time to do it, and easy to find excuses not to do it. But when you finally do, you remember how great it makes you feel. Having sex just once a week can raise your testosterone levels and foster that all-important connection between you and your partner.

That's why, when asked how couples can avoid sex ruts, our first response is always the same: *Just do it!* Make an effort, even if you think you're not in the mood. One of the great things about being a woman is that you may not even be aware of your physical arousal (increased blood flow to the genitals) and don't necessarily experience sexual desire before you have sex. Simply put, desire is the result of sex, not the cause. That means that a woman can "take one for the team" when you think you don't really want sex and still end up having a great time—and possibly an orgasm. For more details, see "The Gift of Sex" on page 284.

It also helps to inject some fun back into your sex life. There's no need for things to be serious and romantic all the time. Back in part 5, we asked you think back to childhood for some very adult inspiration. Here we'd like to remind you of some sexy ways to recapture that sense of playfulness in bed.

PLAY DATE. Every now and then, your sex life needs a change of scenery. So get a sitter and get out of the house. Whether you hightail it to a high-end hotel or a by-the-hour, "no tell" motel is up to you (and your budget). You can even ask your friends with kids to swap child care and use of their home in return for the same. It doesn't really matter, as long as sex and couple time are your goals. Lisa and Harry find that quick getaways like these—even if they only last a few hours—help them reconnect as a couple and make sex the centerpiece of the evening or afternoon, while the novelty of a new location makes things even more exciting.

TOY CHEST. Your kids shouldn't be the only ones with a collection of playthings. Browse online shops together and choose toys you'll both enjoy, such as vibrators, restraints, penis rings, and massage oils. For details on buying and using your new toys, see part 7 of this book.

STORY TIME. Select some books of erotica (try our suggestions on page 203) and read your favorite passages to each other before bed. If you're particularly inspired, try acting out a scene or two.

DRESS UP. Swap your very important but very unsexy roles of "Mommy" and "Daddy" for some decidedly more sensual personas. Refer back to part 7 for role-playing suggestions, or just add a new twist to date night by arriving at a restaurant or bar separately, pretending to be other people (or the people you were when you first met, preparenthood), and getting your flirt on.

RELATIONSHIP ROADBLOCKS

You kid-proof your home, from locks on the cabinets to parental controls on the TV. But what about your relationship? In addition to the problems of finding the time and energy for intimacy, parenthood can have less obvious—but more insidious—effects on your sex life:

PORN PROBLEMS. It's natural for new fathers to use porn to cope with the sex rut that tends to accompany a new baby—many women are so wrapped up in their little one that they don't even notice. That's not always a problem: Masturbation lets your guy blow off a little sexual steam and you don't need to worry about him begging you for sex constantly. But if he starts to spend more time on the computer or with his magazines and DVDs than with you, there's a problem. For advice on dealing with porn dependency, see part 7 of this book.

FLIRTY FRIENDSHIPS. If you're so preoccupied with your kids that you start to lose your own identities, one or both of you may start to look for emotional intimacy outside of your relationship. Who could blame you: Flirting is fun, thrilling, and harmless, right? Well, not exactly. As with porn, e-mail, and instant messaging, social networking sites have made flirty friendships easier than ever to achieve, and soon you may start to rely on your new friend rather than your partner for an emotional connection. If you're concerned that a friendship may be crossing the line, watch for these signs:

- Close friendship and emotional intimacy. A feeling of shared closeness and understanding is one of the early aspects of an emotional affair.

- Secrecy. When you stop sharing certain aspects of the friendship with your partner, and start confiding more in your friend, you're headed toward cheating.

- Sexual attraction. Add a bit of fantasy to the friendship and you've got a recipe for potential disaster: Now you've seen this friend in a sexual light, and your emotional affair could become a physical one.

ian says . . . WHAT YOUR GUY WANTS YOU TO KNOW

Ever wonder what your guy is thinking? As a sex counselor, I'm constantly approached by new dads who have a lot to say about sex and relationships—they just don't always say it to their partners. Here's a peek inside your man's most common thoughts:

"I WANT TO CUDDLE." Even if your partner was never very cuddly before, seeing you with your new baby can make him start to crave the physical and emotional connection that accompanies a simple snuggle. So give him a thirty-second hug—there's no rule that says it has to lead to sex, but it can make you both feel really good.

"I WISH YOU'D INITIATE SEX." Yes, we know that sex can seem like a chore to busy moms, but we're going to keep asking anyway in the hopes that one day soon you'll give in. Sex starts to feel like it's our responsibility, and that can be exhausting in its own way. Every now and then, surprise us with some dirty talk, a secret fantasy, or a pat on the butt. Everyone wants to feel wanted, men included.

"I WANT 'ME' TIME, TOO." Your guy loves spending time with you, in and out of bed. But just as you crave time alone or with your friends, we're dying for a night out with the guys. Please don't make us feel guilty about it: We know we never get to go out and do stuff together; we know we constantly complain about how we just want to spend quality time together (i.e., have sex); and we know we promised you a night at the ballet. But as much as we love you, you're . . . not a guy. New moms need time-outs, and so do new dads. Trade child-care duties with us and we'll return the favor.

"YOU LOOK HOT." You know this, right? Oh, what, you don't? You might suspect your guy is going crazy or losing his eyesight if he thinks you look sexy when you feel dumpy, when your clothes are covered in a fine film of baby puke, and when you haven't showered in two days. And yes, you look awesome after a visit to the salon and when you're wearing that little black

dress. But the truth is, we think you look pretty hot all the time. Men still think about sex at least a hundred times a day, and no one makes us think about it more than our partners.

"IT TURNS ME ON THAT YOU'RE THE MOTHER OF MY CHILD." Sex is all about confidence, right? Well, nothing gives us more of a jolt of pride than to look at you and the kids and think, "Wow, I'm a husband and father now!" And you're partly responsible for that. You, your man, your kids—there's an "us" now, and that can feel amazing.

lisa says . . . HAVING THE BIG TALK

Sex and parenthood don't just mean finding the time for intimacy with your partner—they also mean speaking with your kids about sexuality. It's a conversation that can be filled with embarrassment for you and your child. But the alternative is worse: Kids pick up a lot of misinformation about sex from their friends (and especially from the media) and may have questions but don't know how to ask you about them. I want my daughters to feel comfortable talking to me about everything, including sex, so I've taken a proactive approach to sex ed.

I believe in answering sex-related questions truthfully when children are younger, but only giving them the information they ask for. As kids get older, though, they need more details. When Delilah and Amelia were twelve and nine, a bunch of moms and I brought a sexual educator to my home for a discussion about sex and puberty. We tried to make what could have been an awkward conversation into a fun mother-daughter afternoon, which we all enjoyed. Since then, a lot of our chats about sexuality seem to occur in the car: They feel more at ease because it's not a serious sit-down talk (I'm driving!), and the words just seem to flow more freely and naturally.

I want my girls to feel empowered about their bodies and sexuality. I've tried to make it clear that they can talk to me about anything, including sex, and I encourage you to do the same. After all, if you're not talking to your kids about sex, who is?

try this: THE GIFT OF SEX

Not in the mood for sex? Give it a try anyway—and give your guy the gift of a little sex.

Don't get us wrong: Charity sex isn't the same as pity sex. Instead, it's a way to reestablish a connection with your partner and to make an important investment in your relationship. Think of sex as your favorite charity and sex as a donation to help that cause thrive. Charity sex isn't about meeting someone else's physical needs—it's about meeting your relationship's emotional ones.

There are any number of reasons to engage in charity sex. You might do it because your partner is all wound up from work, and sex relaxes him. You might do it because he's feeling a little down, and sex gives him a boost. Or maybe you do it because—like some forty-one million Americans—you've both gone too many days, weeks, or even *months* without sex. Whatever your motivation, here's how to do it right:

- **Fake it till you make it.** No. We're not advocating fake orgasms. But there's definitely something to be said for putting in a little effort. With charity sex, you may not initially feel as if you're in the mood, but if you start going through the motions, your desire will likely catch up. So start slowly, with intimate touching. Allow *yourself* to enjoy some pleasurable sensations. Try not to think about *anything*—your to-do list; that meeting tomorrow morning—but how it feels when the two of you touch. Before you know it, that offering of charity sex will start to feel like a gift to *both* of you.

- **Take the focus off orgasm.** When you're not in the mood for sex, an orgasm may seem unattainable. And you wonder why you should even bother. But there's a lot to be said for foreplay. So don't fixate too much on the result. Rather, enjoy those delicious caresses and nibbles as they're happening. Stay in the moment—your body may surprise you.

- **Use your brain.** Remember all the reasons you're together. What were things like when they were still new and hot? How have things changed? How can you give back to that relationship? What are you willing to do to bring it back to life?

POP QUIZ

According to the recently released National Survey of Sexual Health and Behavior, which age group is least likely to engage in protected sex?

(A) People ages 18 to 21

(B) People ages 21 to 27

(C) People ages 30 to 40

(D) People age 40 and older

Answer: (D) People age 40 and older. Those irresponsible baby boomers! Haven't they heard the phrase "no glove, no love"? Sure, when you're over forty there's less chance of an unwanted pregnancy, and also more chance of being in a stable committed relationship without the need for protection. But watch out: In our age of Viagra, cougars, and May-December relationships, that age group is more likely than ever to engage in casual sex. Remember, you're never too old to keep a condom in your wallet.

part twelve

SEX:
better
WITH AGE?

At first blush, "aging" and "hot sex" don't exactly seem to go hand in hand. When you think about it, though, it makes sense. It's been said that some things, like fine wine and cheese, only get better with age. And— aches, pains, and gray hairs aside—the passing years can also impart a certain hard-won wisdom and newfound confidence. We're more secure with ourselves, more self-assured about our professional and parenting skills, and more comfortable with our partners and relationships. Is it any wonder, then, that sex can get better, too?

That revelation probably comes as a shock to your younger self. Who, as a teenager, wasn't at least a little bit grossed out by the thought of older people having sex? Of course, back then, "older" probably meant forty (or worse, our parents). Most of us grow up with the idea that sex is something best reserved for the young: If you're old enough to qualify for the senior discount, you're too old to be getting busy.

Once we start to experience aging in earnest, though, we tend to change our minds. Although menopause, low testosterone levels, and other health-related issues can certainly affect your bedroom style, it's more than possible to enjoy a steamy sex life well into your golden years. In fact, research shows that advancing age doesn't have to put a damper on your sexuality: Findings from the large National Social Life, Health, and Aging Project (NSLHAP) found that many Americans remain sexually active well into their seventies and even eighties.

FOXY OVER FIFTY

We're all familiar with the unfair sexual stereotypes of aging men and women: An older man is "distinguished" and "a silver fox," while an older woman is expected to mask her gray hair and wrinkles. Fortunately, that view seems to be changing as baby boomer women hit midlife and beyond. Today you don't have to look much further than the latest issue of *People* to see plenty of gorgeous older women. What makes them so sexy? Yes, they're beautiful, but it's more than that. Compare the self-confidence, wisdom, and life experience of a sixty-year-old with, say, a twenty-year-old, and there's no question as to which woman is more sensual. Older women are more comfortable in their skin, and there's nothing sexier than that. Here are some of our favorite sexy older women:

- Madonna (53)
- Michelle Pfeiffer (53)
- Iman (56)
- Christie Brinkley (57)
- Oprah Winfrey (57)
- Anjelica Huston (60)
- Sigourney Weaver (62)
- Jaclyn Smith (64)
- Cher (65)
- Diane Keaton (65)
- Susan Sarandon (65)
- Goldie Hawn (66)
- Helen Mirren (66)
- Raquel Welch (71)
- Jessica Lange (62)
- Tina Turner (72)
- Jane Fonda (74)
- Sophia Loren (77)
- Joan Collins (78)
- Betty White (90)

25

HORMONES
AND YOUR SEX LIFE

It's clear that the ability to maintain a vibrant sex life into older age depends greatly on our health in general. Natural age-related changes such as shifting hormone levels, as well as chronic conditions that become more likely with time, conspire to make good sex a bit trickier for both men and women. In the NSLHAP study mentioned earlier, researchers found that health, rather than age itself, has more to do with waning sexual activity in older people. The good news: Many of these issues are temporary or manageable—while they may require some flexibility and creativity on your part, they don't have to dictate your sexuality or force you into a sexless relationship.

MENOPAUSE: CH-CH-CHANGES

Menopause—the end of menstruation—is a time of transition, and your sex life is no exception. The ovaries gradually cease functioning and, as a result, levels of estrogen, testosterone, and progesterone drop. This decline in estrogen means less blood flow to your genitals and, in turn, decreased vaginal lubrication. Lower levels of testosterone can affect desire, so you're less motivated to pursue sex. Menopause can also trigger other causes of low libido: You may struggle with insomnia, irritability, depression, and hot flashes, none of which exactly make you feel in the mood. You might feel less feminine and sexual or dissatisfied with your body in general, as well.

But there are benefits to menopause, too. Some women feel even more sensual and find that their sex drive actually increases over time. According to the results of a recent survey by Good in Bed, the quality and frequency of women's orgasms improves with age, too. Plus, you no longer have to worry about contraception and pregnancy, which can give you a new sense of freedom. Where "The Change" was once viewed as the end of a woman's sexual self, today we've got a seemingly endless array of sexy "older woman" role models, from Susan Sarandon to Tina Turner (see "Foxy Over Fifty" on page 289). They're living proof that it's more than possible to be smoking hot, well beyond midlife.

Of course, that may be cold comfort if you're smack in the middle of menopausal symptoms and the sexual side effects they can produce. The key to staying sexually active is to work with these changes, not against them. Whether you choose to use hormone replacement therapy or other treatment is up to you and your doctor. For the most part, though, you can address sexual symptoms with a few key approaches.

VAGINAL DRYNESS. The hormonal changes of menopause can thin and dry out already delicate vaginal tissues, making sex uncomfortable and even painful for nearly 40 percent of postmenopausal women. Use the tips in part 5 of this book to select a lubricant that works well for you and your partner, and use it every time you are intimate, not just during intercourse. Choose sexual positions such as "woman on top" that allow you to control the angle, depth, and speed of penetration and avoid those (such as rear entry) that involve deep thrusting.

LOW LIBIDO. Those fluctuating hormones can also dampen desire. Boost your sex drive with the advice in part 9 of this book: Make intimacy (kissing, hugging, cuddling, and touching) a priority, even if you and your partner don't have sex. Practice stress management techniques that help you relax and unwind, an important aspect of female sexual desire and arousal. Read a piece of erotica or watch a sexy movie with your partner, and give each other sensual massages.

AROUSAL DIFFICULTIES. Reduced blood flow to the genitals may make physical arousal more difficult for you, even if you're mentally turned on. Experiment with vibrators, female arousal gels, and other products that increase blood flow and stimulate the clitoris. For more tips, check out part 9.

IS YOUR MAN IN MENOPAUSE?

Women aren't the only ones who experience a transition in hormones, health, and sex as they age. Men face their own challenges, too. Male-specific age-related issues are largely driven by testosterone—or, more accurately, dwindling levels of it. As you learned earlier, this hormone is critical for a satisfying sex

IS IT ED OR LOW T?

Many men confuse andropause with erectile dysfunction (ED), because they often occur around the same time. These men often turn to an ED medication, such as Viagra, to improve their erectile ability, which works temporarily in most cases. However, as men get older, the gap between desire and arousal widens and many men become deeply disappointed when Viagra doesn't give them the desire to have sex. That's because many of these men are actually dealing with low testosterone, not ED—and Viagra doesn't boost testosterone levels. In other words, they don't have a problem with physical arousal, but with mental arousal. If your guy is grappling with the desire for sex—or if Viagra doesn't seem to work for him—he should consider a trip to his doctor to check his testosterone levels. For more information about ED, see part 10 of this book.

life in both men and women, although it plays a larger role in guys. Just like women, as a man advances into his forties he experiences a progressive decline in hormone levels—in this case, testosterone. If testosterone drops low enough, it can be a sign that a man is in "male menopause." Technically known as andropause, it affects about five million American men and can have a very real impact on a guy's mood, health, and sex life.

Low testosterone doesn't always signal a problem: There's a huge range in what is considered normal for testosterone. Levels of this hormone fluctuate greatly throughout the day—they're highest in the morning—and even during different seasons. Life itself can also affect testosterone. When a guy enters a steady relationship, for example, his levels tend to drop somewhat, and then decrease even further when he has small children. (This may be Nature's sneaky way of trying to ensure that dads remain monogamous and supportive of their offspring.) Interestingly, any type of competition, from a friendly game of tag football to an attempt to get you into bed, can change a man's testosterone levels to prepare him for the challenge. Research suggests that if he succeeds in his quest to win, his testosterone will spike by about 20 percent—but if he fails, his testosterone could *drop* by as much as 90 percent. Even more complicated, two men of the same age may have exactly the same testosterone level but feel very different, physically, emotionally, and sexually.

In general, though, lower levels of testosterone are apt to make a guy feel moody, irritable, and depressed. They can also raise his risk of heart disease and lower his bone density, making him more prone to injury. And as you might imagine, decreased testosterone can hurt his sex life, mainly by making it more difficult for him to get and stay aroused. Testosterone is truly the hormone that stokes the flames of desire—and without enough of it, his libido may suffer.

Don't make assumptions, though: Andropause isn't the same as a midlife crisis, and not all men who experience the inevitable decline in testosterone that accompanies aging have andropause. If you think your partner might be

ian says . . . HOW MASTURBATION SAPS HIS MOJO

I've said it before in this book and I'll say it again: Masturbation is a good thing. It helps us get in touch with our sexuality (literally), helps us learn what we like, and is an important part of a healthy relationship. For women, masturbating regularly can help keep vaginal tissues moist by promoting blood flow to the genitals. For men, though, masturbation is a double-edged sword. While self-pleasuring can keep blood flowing to the penis, it doesn't always have a positive effect on a guy's sex life.

The problem occurs when men in their forties and older keep masturbating like they're still in their twenties. What used to be typical guy behavior—get off to some porn earlier in the day, hook up with his partner later on—is now a real issue. A man who's, say, forty-five, just doesn't have the same refractory period as a twenty-five-year-old man. It takes longer for him to recover after an orgasm and get an erection again. If he's already masturbated, he may have nothing left to give by the time he tries to have sex with a woman. It's not a problem with low desire or erectile dysfunction—he's simply squandered his mojo.

That's why I usually suggest that older men refrain from masturbating if they plan to have sex with a partner within the next few days. If you sense this is an issue for your guy, don't demand that he give up porn or stop masturbating, but do ask him to save his energy for you—and then suggest all the steamy ways you'll make it worth his while.

coping with andropause, remember that it's a medical condition that a physician must diagnose with a blood test. If the test confirms that he has low levels of testosterone, he may want to boost the hormone on his own with nondrug approaches: Chronic stress, a boring routine, feeling unappreciated and purposeless at work, being unemployed, a lack of physical activity and exercise, and even some cholesterol-lowering medications can all sink testosterone. Your guy should try to keep a regular schedule of both aerobic exercise and weight training, get proper levels of sleep, manage stress, get appropriate levels of zinc in his diet, and do things that help him experience a sense of accomplishment and success regularly.

If your man has followed all these measures, but still has low testosterone, he may want to consider asking his doctor for pharmaceutical help. Just as there are various hormone replacement therapies for women, there's also testosterone replacement therapy for men, which is available as a skin patch, gel, and injection. Because testosterone therapy can have a number of side effects, including decreased sperm production and an enlarged prostate, men should never use it without a doctor's supervision.

Whatever you and your partner decide to do, we want to stress that just because a man may be past his testosterone peak doesn't mean he's past his sexual peak. He might not be having sex the way he did at age twenty or thirty—you probably aren't, either—but that's not necessarily a sign that something's wrong. Once you know what's going on and realize that hormonal decline can affect men, too, you can take a proactive lead in talking about it with him. That's important, because when a man embraces a deeper intimacy and opens himself up to a different experience of sex, the passage of time can bring many rewards.

26

SHARED
CHALLENGES

the hormonal changes that affect men and women can have a big impact on our sex lives, but so can a slew of other issues related to age. From health problems like heart disease and arthritis, to emotionally charged transitions such as a newly empty nest and retirement, you and your partner can both find your-selves coping with additional challenges to a healthy sex life. But that doesn't mean that things have to cool off altogether. By working together, you can learn how to adjust for these obstacles so that you both stay satisfied.

WHY YOUR HEALTH MATTERS

A steady diet of Big Macs, Diet Coke, and *Project Runway* marathons can seem benign when we're younger, but these bad habits can add up as we age, clog-ging our arteries, packing on the pounds, and leading to a greater risk of problems including high cholesterol, high blood pressure, heart disease, and diabetes, all of which can impair blood flow to the genitals in both men and women. With age comes an increased incidence of other conditions—arthritis, bladder control issues, and prostate problems, for example—that aren't directly responsible for sexual dys-function but can quash your feelings of desire and arousal. Plus, some medications

try this: EASY INTIMACY

Sex doesn't have to be all about acrobatic positions and the latest toys. That's all great, of course, but you can have mind-blowing sex simply by increasing the intimate gestures you and your partner bring to the table (or, more likely, the bed). Some experts believe that maintaining eye contact during sex can lead to greater intimacy, because it encourages you to have sex using both your heart and your mind, not just with your genitals. And, if you've been practicing the thirty-second hugs described in part 1, you already know all about the positive, oxytocin-boosting impact of physical intimacy. (If you skipped that section, get back there and get to work!) This exercise is aimed at amping up your sexual connection with your partner—no flexible hamstrings or props required.

Warm up by engaging in some thirty-second hugs throughout the day. We find that such hugs help us feel closer to our partners, less stressed, and more willing to "go there" sexually later on. Once you're ready for bed, melt into each other and hold on tight. We're talking longer than thirty seconds now—maybe a few minutes. It probably will feel emotionally awkward but physically comforting. Just when you're ready to pull away, hang on a little longer. Then take a deep breath and get ready for the next step.

Gaze into each other's eyes as you turn each other on by kissing and touching each other. Don't look away, even if you feel uncomfortable. Stop worrying about your orgasm or his, and simply focus on what you see in each other's eyes. When you do climax, keep those eyes locked. This heightened intimate connection should send your pleasure through the roof and may linger long after your orgasms have come and gone.

used to treat these and other age-related health issues can decrease libido, delay your orgasm and his ejaculation, and otherwise affect sexuality. These problems affect men and women, but their impact on men's sexuality may be more obvious: Decreased blood flow to the penis means an inability to get and maintain an erection. In fact, the large NSLHAP study found that 64 percent of women and 55 percent of men cite the male partner's physical health as the number-one reason for a lack of sexual activity in their relationship. Men and women alike can benefit from our tips for sexual fitness in part 3 of this book. You can find plenty of advice for preventing and treating a variety of male and female sexual issues—including erectile dysfunction, difficulties climaxing, and low libido—in parts 5 and 7.

CHANGE OF LIFE: MOVING ON, TOGETHER

Most couples approach the departure of their last child from the nest with a mix of excitement and trepidation. On the one hand, you've got the house to your-selves to use as your sexual playground (why, hello again, dining room table!). On the other, once the kids are gone, many couples find that they have little left in common except parenthood—an empty nest is often a trigger for divorce. That's also true of retirement: All that constant togetherness can be irritating, especially if one partner has already been at home for a while.

But there's a positive side to these changes, too: When you approach transi-tions as opportunities to reconnect, your relationship (and sexual) satisfaction can improve. A study in the November 2008 issue of *Psychological Science* found that women's marital satisfaction tends to increase after their children have left home, not just because they have more free time but because they enjoy their partner more. And a 2008 survey by the AARP showed that 78 percent of couples enjoy just as much sex as they did before retirement and 38 percent say they're even more romantic. Take the time to really reinvest in your relation-ship—including your sex life—and enjoy the spoils.

REMINISCE. What first attracted you to each other? While his rock-hard abs may have softened, his wicked sense of humor probably hasn't. Think back to the beginning of your relationship and enjoy those same qualities now. Research suggests that acting like strangers on a first date can reignite attraction; so can a little role-playing—which is easier than ever with your new free time and privacy.

FAN THE FLAMES. Our biggest sex organ is the brain, right? Don't let your exit from the working world leave you with little to discuss with your partner. Ward off boredom by flexing your intellectual muscles: Volunteer, get a hobby, take an adult ed class, start crossing things off of a dream "bucket" list. When your life is thrilling outside the bedroom, your sex life will get more stimulating, too.

In the same regard, using your brain can also help spice things up between the sheets. Our libidos may lag as we get older, but the "second honeymoon" that results from retirement or an empty nest can actually give your sex drive a lift. Talk about your fantasies, read erotica, or watch a sexy movie together. Keeping the communication flowing and your desire and arousal will follow.

MIX IT UP. Even if you look like a twenty-five-year-old, your body—and stamina—is still different now. If *Kama Sutra*–inspired positions seem more like an amusing way to pull a muscle and end up in the emergency room than the gateway to hot sex, it's time to start making some adjustments. Got a bad back? Forego the missionary position for more comfortable options like side by side or spooning, for example. Variety helps, too: If you enjoy a wider range of sexual activities in you sex life, you'll have more options for pleasure at your disposal. Recognize that "sex" doesn't *have* to equal "intercourse," and you'll have a lot more options for pleasure. Kissing, cuddling, touching, oral sex, manual stimulation, and vibrators and other sex toys never go out of style. In fact, research shows that people who remain sexually active as they age find ways to stay that way, despite limitations: About half of couples under age seventy-five still engage in oral sex, while half of men and a quarter of women still masturbate, whether or not they have a partner. Think in terms of what you *can* do sexually, not what you can't.

LOOK ON THE BRIGHT SIDE. Just because sex isn't what it was twenty years ago doesn't mean it's worse. Focus on the aspects of your sex life that improve with age: A younger man may have stronger erections, for instance, but an older guy tends to have better control. Plus, you both know each other's bodies, you've perfected your technique, and you may feel less inhibited than you did in the past.

---

good idea: BEST SEX TOYS FOR OLDER LOVERS

Please don't dismiss vibrators and other toys as props for younger couples only. These products can be a huge help for getting and staying aroused at all ages, but they're particularly useful for postmenopausal women and their partners. Vibrators, especially those that provide clitoral stimulation, can jump-start a flagging sex life: They promote blood flow to the genitals, boost arousal, and can give your guy (and his penis) a much-needed break. But not all toys are created equal. Here's what to look for when shopping for them.

- **Flexibility.** Just as kitchen utensils and other tools are now available in senior-friendly variations, sex toys are becoming more ergonomic, too. Look for those that can be used hands-free—vibes shaped like eggs, bullets, and computer mice are good options—or that can bend and twist to allow for physical limitations.

- **Strength.** As we age, it can take longer to get where we want to go sexually. Your vibrator should be able to take a licking and keep on ticking. Check reviews to find those with longer battery lives.

- **Speed.** Many older women find that vibes with stronger vibrations can help them get aroused more easily. Choose models with multiple speeds so you can adjust your pleasure level accordingly.

Whatever toys you buy, be sure to use plenty of lube—older vaginal tissues are delicate and tend to require a bit more moisture. For more information on senior sex, check out *Better Than I Ever Expected* and *Naked at Our Age* by Joan Price.

THE TEN-STEP
SEX WORKOUT

We've said it before: great sex is like any other part of a healthy lifestyle—it helps you feel good, both physically and emotionally. We all know that a balanced diet and a well-rounded approach to exercise are optimal for well-being: Nutritionists recommend filling your plate with a variety of foods, from brightly colored produce, to whole grains, to lean proteins. Personal trainers tell us that we should try different activities—lifting weights, doing yoga, hitting the elliptical—to work our various muscles.

Why not view your sex life similarly? Sure, sex is sex. But there's a whole range of intriguing options under that broad label:

- There's good old comfort sex—the "if it ain't broke, don't fix it" approach that many long-term couples take.

- There's gentle, tender lovemaking.

- There's no-holds-barred sex for the sake of sex.

- There's the frantic quickie.

- There's long, languorous sex that plays on all the senses.

- There's playful, lighthearted sex.

- There's solo sex that puts all the attention on the person who knows how to please you best—you! As Woody Allen said in *Annie Hall*, "Don't knock masturbation, it's sex with someone I love."

These are just a few of the many scenarios you can choose from every time you have sex. Yet if you and your partner are like most long-term couples, nine times out of ten, you probably go the safe, familiar comfort sex route.

There's nothing wrong with that. But why not use this book as an opportunity to step outside the box a bit? Whether you've read it from cover to cover or skipped around to the sections that interest you most, you've undoubtedly discovered a bunch of fun, sexy ideas that sparked curiosity in you or your partner. So put what you've learned to good use. We've compiled some of our favorite "sexercises" into a ten-step program that you and your partner can complete at your own pace. Want to shake things up in bed? Looking for a fun way to blow off some sexual steam? Need new ideas to help make the most of date night? We've got you covered.

There's no need to follow these exercises in order, and there's no recommended time frame. You could try one scenario a week, or, if you're feeling ambitious, do the whole program in just ten days. Or you could turn to these ideas throughout the year, anytime you're looking for ways to get out of a sex rut or spice things up between the sheets. There's no right or wrong way to use the exercises. Just keep an open mind and an open heart—and have fun!

SEXERCISE #1:
SOLO MISSION

BEST WHEN: You're in a long-distance relationship; you or your partner are coping with a low libido; you're in a sex rut.

HOW TO: Research shows that orgasm lights up all parts of the brain, including those associated with memory. Orgasm plays a powerful role in the reward centers of the brain, so it makes sense that the more we associate that positive reward with a particular person, or memory of a person, the more we reinforce our overall relationship with that person. It also stands to reason that masturbating with your partner in mind might increase your feelings of love and desire toward that person via the reward of orgasm.

Even if you can't have sex with your partner—maybe you're on opposite coasts right now, or one of you is grappling with a low sex drive—you can enjoy a sense of closeness. For this exercise, we'd like you to skip anything you usually use to turn yourself on during masturbation. That means porn (Internet, magazines, movies), erotica, romance novels, reruns of *True Blood* . . . It should just be you, some lube, a toy if you like, and your lusty thoughts about your partner. Think back to a time when you had amazing sex with each other. Really go there: Where were you? What did the setting look and smell like? What did it feel like to touch him and to be touched? As you caress yourself now, let the memories of sex with your partner take hold and bring you over the edge.

The concept of this exercise might seem a little strange: After all, you're indulging in some solo self-pleasure. But the truth is that by conjuring up your partner during this pleasurable time, you can create a positive association that links the thought of him with sensual feelings and vice versa. This exercise should help you feel closer to your guy and may even help lift you out of a rut by putting you in the mood for sex with him.

SEXERCISE #2: SENSUAL SEX

BEST WHEN: You want to reconnect with your partner; you have some extra time.

HOW TO: Sex should involve all of our senses—it's *sensual,* after all. Too often, though, we don't take full advantage of these sensations. For this exercise, we'd like you to slow things down. Stop and smell the roses, if you will. Start by preparing your bedroom to appeal to the senses: Light some scented candles, make the bed with clean sheets (try satin or a soft, higher-thread-count cotton), and play a selection of sexy songs on your stereo or iPod. Take turns feeding each other from a spread of yummy treats like strawberries and chocolate. For an added kick, don a blindfold à la *9 ½ Weeks* and guess what delicacies your partner is using to tempt you.

Then focus on the sense of touch. Collect items that you think would feel interesting against your skin—silk scarves, soft blankets, feathers, massage tools . . . If S&M intrigues, include some supplies such as a paddle or riding crop. Now experiment with different types of touch: To play with temperature, use the hot wax from a massage candle on some of your partner's more sensitive areas, like the small of his back or his nipples, before moving on to the rest of his body. For contrast, grab some ice cubes from the freezer and glide one slowly over your partner's skin, tracing it over his body. Now switch places. If you want to dabble in pain and pleasure, try spanking each other (either with an open palm or a paddle), starting slow in order to ensure arousal, and then building up in both speed and pressure. Follow up with a gentle massage. Whatever you choose, you'll both likely discover new opportunities for arousal.

SEXERCISE #3:
NEW MOVES

BEST WHEN: You're bored with the same old, same old.

HOW TO: Is the missionary position like second nature to you? Do you find your-selves slipping into the same familiar arrangement every time you have inter-course? Maybe it's time to give some new positions a test drive. Tonight, make an agreement to experiment with one or more different sexual positions that you haven't tried before. Flip through this book for ideas that strike your fancy, whether that's a variation of woman on top such as reverse cowgirl, an orgasm-friendly position such as the coital alignment technique (CAT), or a move such as doggy-style that gives your guy a great view. Need more inspiration? You can find playing cards, games, and books (including the *Kama Sutra*) filled with position ideas. There are even smartphone apps that offer a new position every day. While you might still return to your same old comfortable positions most of the time, this exercise can help you discover a few new favorites, too.

SEXERCISE #4:
THE FAST AND THE FURIOUS

BEST WHEN: You're short on time but long on passion; you're in a sex rut.

HOW TO: Finally! The kids are napping, your houseguests just turned in for the night, you're on a lunch break—and you're in the mood. Or maybe just the opposite is true: You feel like you never have any quality "couple" time these days. You've barely got a moment to kiss each other good night, let alone indulge in a lengthy lovemaking session. And we all know what happens then: The longer you go without sex, the less you want it.

Fortunately, the opposite is true, too. Sex begets sex, and sometimes all you need to jump-start things in the bedroom is to get hot and heavy, even if it's just for a few smoldering minutes. That's why we're big fans of the quickie—the quickie done *right,* that is. We've talked about the basics earlier in this book, but it bears repeating here: You want to build arousal throughout the day so that by the time you actually attempt intercourse, you're both ready to explode. So start early with a long, deep kiss good-bye before work. Keep ramping up arousal during the day with saucy e-mails and texts, phone messages promising what's to come later, and some passionate groping back at home. See how far you can go while your clothes are still on and no one's looking. Later, meet up at a predetermined spot—the bathroom, say, or the laundry room, or yes, even the bedroom—for a fast and furious hookup. Chances are that you'll both be so turned on that no foreplay will be necessary.

SEXERCISE #5: STOP AND GO

BEST WHEN: You've got all night; you want to explore your potential for multiple orgasms; you want to extend your sexual staying power.

HOW TO: This exercise is the polar opposite of The Fast and the Furious, with one distinct thing in common: Here, you're going to take your own sweet time with sex, but you'll still aim for a pleasure-packed climax—or two, or three, or more. It's all about resisting the urge to race your partner to the orgasmic finish line. Instead, we want you to keep bringing each other to the edge and then pull back.

Get comfy and lock that bedroom door (this is a good exercise to save for when the kids are at a sleepover or for when you and your sweetie are staying at a hotel). Don't forget to grab some lube—you're going to need it! Now, start with some foreplay. Try the erotic massage described in part 5 of this book, spending plenty of time and attention on all your favorite body parts. Then move on to some manual and oral stimulation. Women can experiment with some of the different hand and blow job techniques from part 5. Men can slowly explore their partner's vulva and clitoris with fingers and tongue. You can include a toy like a vibrator here, too, but be careful! We don't want you to climax just yet, so keep the vibrations on low and set it aside if you feel yourself approaching orgasm.

When you're both ready for intercourse, keep up the slow pace. When your partner first penetrates you, he should keep his thrusts shallow, remaining close to the opening of you vagina, which allows your orgasm to build slowly. If your guy feels like he's going to climax, he can pull out for a bit, slow down, use the perpendicular penis positions described in part 10. Eventually, though, he should flip you on top, which is the best position for you to achieve multiple orgasms. But women aren't the only ones who have the ability to climax more than once. With practice, men may be able to experience multiple orgasms as well. By concentrating on his breathing, and keeping things slow and steady, he may be able to feel the pleasurable waves of orgasm even if he doesn't ejaculate. Whether you end up having five orgasms or one, this exercise can help sex last all night long.

SEXERCISE #6: TRADING FAVORS

BEST WHEN: You want to focus all your attention on your partner—and receive the same in kind.

HOW TO: We give a lot of attention to the intercourse aspect of sex, but the fact is that there are many different pathways to orgasm and not all of them require a penis in a vagina. Tonight we want you to take a different journey, one that allows you and your partner to take turns giving and receiving pleasure. Start by inviting your partner to relax on your bed as you give him an erotic massage. Next, pour some lube on your palms (give them a good rub together to warm it up) and try out one or more of the hand job scenarios described in part 7 of this book. Take your time as you experiment to see which moves turn him on the most.

You could bring him to climax right now—but where's the fun in that? Instead, let him suffer alone for a few tortuous moments. Maybe you'll take things a step further and secure his wrists with handcuffs or ties and slip a blindfold over his eyes to prevent him from seeing the action. And what's coming next? Well, him, if he plays his cards right! After applying more lube (flavored, if you like), use your tongue to trace the lines of his body, from his chest down to his penis and testicles. Play around with the oral sex ideas mentioned in part 5 until you find one that floats his boat. Enjoy his climax—you're up next.

SEXERCISE #7:
SHOW OFF

BEST WHEN: You want to step outside the box—and your bedroom.

HOW TO: Too much PDA (public display of affection) might gross you out, but many of us get a thrill at the idea of being caught having sex, even if the reality of the situation would be mortifying. If you've ever wanted to dabble in exhibitionism, now's your chance. Of course, everyone's boundaries are different: What might make you all hot and bothered might make your guy skittish. Thankfully, there's a wide range of ways to get your exhibitionist kicks—no embarrassment necessary.

Tonight, step outside your comfort zone by stepping outside the bedroom. If you're nervous about leaving home, you don't need to. Declare the boudoir off-limits and start exploring the rest of your house. Maybe you'll clear off the dining room table, or get busy on your screened-in porch, or try the laundry room and discover if the vibrations from the washing machine add an extra sexual thrill. Do it in front of a window (this works best if you don't have close neighbors), or in front of a full-length mirror.

Craving more adventure? Do it at your parents' house during a holiday visit. Make out in your parked car. Flirt like crazy during a dinner date, or get frisky in a darkened movie theater. If you decide to go all the way, scope out private places where you're less likely to get busted: a secluded alley, an empty beach, a locked restroom. Remember, the *idea* of getting caught is hot. The reality of a public indecency charge? Not so much.

SEXERCISE #8:
TANTRIC SEX

BEST WHEN: You want to take the focus off orgasm; you have the time to slow down and enjoy each other.

HOW TO: Feeling a bit out of touch with your partner? Has it been too long since you really, *really* made love? A steamy session of tantric sex may be just the thing you need to reconnect with each other. This is also a great exercise if you've been having difficulty climaxing, because it takes the focus off of orgasm and allows you both to enjoy pleasure for pleasure's sake.

As you learned earlier in this book, tantra itself is a religious philosophy in which practitioners seek to harness the divine power that they believe flows through the universe as a way to attain their goals. Tantric sex, or the use of sexual intercourse as a form of meditation, is just one small aspect of tantra. Tantric sex can have big benefits: It can help you and your partner feel more attuned to each other and may make your sexual sessions longer, more intense, and more satisfying.

Before you start, though, it's a good idea to begin with some yoga, which can increase flexibility, reduce stress, strengthen pelvic floor (PC) muscles, and has been shown to improve sexual function. Take a class or two with your guy to get in shape—consider it foreplay, if you will. Then, when you're ready, make sure you have some time to devote to sex. As with some of the other "sexercises" here, this is a great time to send your kids to Grandma's house or to splurge on a hotel room.

Do what you can to unwind, whether that means lighting some candles, playing soft music, showering together, giving each other massages, sharing some wine, or all of the above. Next, sit across from each other in bed and gaze into each other's eyes as you try to sync your breathing with your partner's. After about five or ten minutes, start touching each other, all the while talking about what feels food. Concentrate on giving your partner pleasure (he should do the same). Keep up the eye contact and breathing. Now, slowly move into intercourse, exercising your PC muscles to keep your orgasm at bay (see page 149 for details). If you feel yourself approaching climax, slow things down even more and take some deep breaths. Hold off as long as you can. Whether or not you do finally climax, the road you take to get there will be paved with pleasure.

SEXERCISE #9:
PLAY TIME

BEST WHEN: You want to spice things up; you need a little extra help dealing with sexual arousal issues.

HOW TO: Kids have their toys; why shouldn't you? Sex doesn't always have to be all intensity and seduction. There's nothing wrong with a little fun in bed—and one of the best ways to lighten things up is by introducing some playthings into the mix. But toys can have some serious benefits, too: If you're facing arousal difficulties or have trouble reaching orgasm through intercourse alone, a vibrator can be your (and your partner's) best friend. Penis rings keep blood flow trapped in the penis, which, when used sparingly, can help strengthen a man's erection. And props like handcuffs and other restraints can spice up the "sex on demand" aspect of trying to conceive. Take a look back through part 7 of this book for suggestions for choosing and using a variety of toys, then put your selections to good use tonight.

SEXERCISE #10:
MEMORY LANE

BEST WHEN: Your relationship could use a jump start; you want to feel those heady hormones of first lust all over again.

HOW TO: We began this "workout" with an exercise designed to reignite your passion for your partner, even when you're alone. What better way to complete the program than with a scenario that plays on that passion while you're together?

As you learned earlier in this book, newness and novelty trigger the release of the potent brain chemicals dopamine and norepinephrine, both of which play a key role in sexual arousal. When we are first falling in love with someone, just the thought of that person makes us pleasantly jittery. But later, as we move through the relationship cycle into deeper attachment, this is generally replaced by a sense of comfort—that's why falling asleep reading the latest best-seller now seems just as appealing as engaging in a steamy make-out session. So you've got to re-create that sense of newness that made it so hot at the beginning.

Start things off by taking a mental stroll down Memory Lane. Do you remember the time you first locked eyes with him? Can you remember those heady beginning days, where just a light brush of skin on skin sent lightning rushing through your body? You're about to discover that excitement all over again. Flip back to part 6 of this book for some sexy role-playing ideas. One that's been shown to work well at fanning the flames of lust in long-term couples is to pretend to be strangers.

Head out separately to a previously agreed-upon pickup spot, like a bar, club, or restaurant, perhaps slightly altering your appearance with new or different clothing. When you see your partner, approach him and offer to buy him a drink. Exchange fake names, and begin chatting and flirting as you add subtle forms of touch—a hand around the waist, a brush of the knee—to tease each other. Put some effort into the seduction. Finally, invite your partner back to your place. Not only is this hookup pretty much a sure thing, but your make-believe lust will likely translate into some very real passion.

PARTING WORDS

now that you've completed the "Sex Workout," you should be in great shape—emotionally, physically, and sexually. Whether you're a thrill seeker or a comfort creature, whether you're in a long-term relationship or are wading back into the dating pool, whether you're digging yourself out of a sex rut or are just looking for ideas to spice things up, we hope you've gleaned some new tips from this book. If we've helped you learn how to communicate better with your partner, or to cope with sexual issues, or to understand and appreciate each other's body, or to discover new pathways to pleasure, we've accomplished our goal. Remember, sex can be a lot of things—hot, dirty, languorous, blissful, intense, emotional—but it should always be fun. So relax, enjoy, and have a blast!

PHOTO CREDITS

Photo on page x courtesy of Emily A. Miller.

Photo on page xi courtesy of Lois Rinna.